OXFORD MEDICAL OUTLINE SERIES

PERIPHERAL
VASCULAR DISEASES
(ANGIOLOGY)

SAUL S. SAMUELS, A.M., M.D.

CONSULTING VASCULAR SURGEON, LONG BEACH HOSPITAL, LONG BEACH, NEW
YORK; ATTENDING VASCULAR SURGEON, BROOKLYN HOSPITAL FOR THE AGED;
CHIEF OF THE DEPARTMENT OF PERIPHERAL ARTERIAL DISEASES, STUYVESANT
POLYCLINIC HOSPITAL, NEW YORK; FELLOW IN SURGERY, NEW YORK ACADEMY
OF MEDICINE; MEMBER OF COMMITTEE ON SURGERY, NEW YORK DIABETES
ASSOCIATION

OXFORD UNIVERSITY PRESS
LONDON   NEW YORK   TORONTO

PREFACE

In previous years the subject of peripheral vascular diseases was divided indiscriminately among various specialties in medicine and surgery. As a result, insufficient emphasis was placed upon the subject as a whole, leading to a confused classification and a correspondingly inadequate presentation. In some hospitals cases of gangrene of the extremities were assigned haphazardly to the general surgeon, the orthopedist and to the internist merely because diabetes mellitus was also present. In many instances the patient was considered a fit subject for the physical therapist. Many cases of thrombo-angiitis obliterans were held to be within the sphere of the dermatologist who was also given the responsibility for Raynaud's disease and scleroderma.

It is only recently that the profession has become cognizant of the fact that there are so many hitherto unrecognized details of diagnosis and treatment applicable to the peripheral vascular diseases that they necessarily require the attention of someone who has the time and desire to concentrate more effort and attention to these cases. As a result a new specialty has been spontaneously developed which, while unique in many respects, is not very much different from some of the other special branches of medicine and surgery that have been recognized through sheer necessity. As in ophthalmology and gynecology, which require acquaintance with medicine and surgery, so with peripheral vascular diseases one must be thoroughly grounded in internal medicine as well as general surgery to do justice to this field.

In the organic arterial diseases of the extremities one may proceed to only a limited extent in the treatment and management by the utilization of internal medicine alone. When the elements of gangrene and infection enter the picture, surgical training is also a requisite for the successful supervision of the patient. This is particularly true when the question of amputation arises, both in the sense of indications for the operation and performance of the amputation. This lack of training in both fields necessitates a sharp division in management followed by the placing of surgical re-

[iii]

sponsibility upon the shoulders of one whose interest in the case may be purely that of a technician who amputates the limb at the behest of the internist. Growing experience in the field of peripheral vascular diseases brings out the necessity of assigning the entire responsibility to one individual, expertly trained in both medical and surgical phases of the subect, if progress in this field is to be made along present lines with a reduction in the number of cases requiring amputation and in the mortality rate. These ideals can be achieved not only by adherence to this broad outlook but also by instituting a thorough grounding in the general principles of diagnosis and treatment that must be inculcated in the minds of the advanced medical student, the interne and the general practitioner. Sufficient emphasis must be placed upon these principles so that the aspirant in this field shall not be misled into the easy and sometimes lucrative path of the mechanical gadget that purports to cure any and all forms of vascular disease.

As a contribution to the furtherance of this principle, this outline is offered to the student and graduate physician with the hope that it will stimulate further interest in every phase of peripheral vascular diseases with the realization that this subject comprises more than the mere application of a machine or an injection to the solution of the problem. In the knowledge that the comparative novelty of the specialty carries with it many new and controversial ideas, both in diagnosis and treatment, I have attempted to expound those principles which a vast personal experience in private and hospital practice has demonstrated to be sound and workable.

I would like to acknowledge the assistance of Miss Sidonia Reissman and Miss Harriet Shilin in the preparation of the manuscript.

S. S. S.

CONTENTS

ANATOMY OF THE BLOOD VESSELS
OF THE EXTREMITIES

Arteries of the Lower Extremities

A. The Common Iliac Arteries.

1. These are branches of the abdominal aorta. They are about two inches long and divide opposite the intervertebral disc between the last lumbar vertebra and the sacrum into:

   a. The internal iliac artery which supplies the contents of the pelvis and

   b. The external iliac artery which becomes the femoral artery at a point beneath Poupart's ligament, midway between the anterior superior spine of the ilium and symphysis pubis.

   c. The femoral artery which passes down the inner side of the thigh to the opening in the adductor magnus at the junction of the middle and lower thirds of the thigh where it becomes the popliteal artery. The branches of the femoral artery are:

      (1) Superficial epigastric.
      (2) Superficial circumflex iliac.
      (3) Superficial external pudic.
      (4) Deep external pudic.
      (5) Muscular.
      (6) Deep femoral.
      (7) Anastomotica magna.

   d. The popliteal artery originates at the termination of the femoral artery at the opening of the adductor magnus muscle, passes downward and outward behind the knee joint to the lower border of the popliteus muscle where it divides into the anterior and posterior tibial arteries. Branches of the popliteal artery are:

      (1) The superior and inferior muscular branches.
      (2) Cutaneous branches.
      (3) Internal superior articular.

(4) Azygos articular.

(5) Internal and external.

e. The anterior tibial artery originates at the bifurcation of the popliteal artery at the lower border of the popliteus muscle, proceeds forward between the heads of the tibialis posticus muscle and through the opening above the upper border of the interosseous membrane to the deep part of the front of the leg to the front of the ankle joint where it becomes the dorsalis pedis artery. The branches of the anterior tibial artery are:

(1) Anterior and posterior recurrent tibial.

(2) Superior fibular.

(3) Muscular.

(4) Internal and external malleolar.

f. The posterior tibial artery proceeds downward from the lower border of the popliteus muscle along the medial side of the leg to the fossa between the internal and external plantar arteries. Its branches are:

(1) Peroneal.

(2) Nutrient.

(3) Muscular.

(4) Cutaneous.

(5) Communicating.

(6) Internal calcaneal.

(7) Malleolar cutaneous.

g. The dorsalis pedis artery, the continuation of the anterior tibial artery, passes forward from the ankle along the medial side of the foot to the first intermetatarsal space where it divides into the dorsalis hallucis artery and a communicating branch. The branches of the dorsalis pedis artery are:

(1) Cutaneous.

(2) Tarsal.

(3) Metatarsal and dorsal interosseous.

(4) Dorsalis hallucis.

(5) Communicating artery.

h. The internal plantar artery is a termination of the posterior tibial artery which passes forward along the inner side of the foot. It gives off digital and cutaneous branches.

i. The external plantar artery is another termination of the posterior tibial artery which passes outward and forward to the base of the fifth metatarsal bone. It anastomoses with a communicating branch of the dorsalis pedis and gives off digital and perforating branches.

Veins of the Lower Extremities

A. Main Superficial Veins of the Leg.

1. The internal or long saphenous vein begins at the medial side of the dorsum of the foot ascending anteriorly to the internal malleolus along the medial side of the leg to the knee where it passes posteriorly to the inner condyle of the femur along the medial side of the thigh passing through the saphenous opening, where it joins the femoral vein about an inch and a half below Poupart's ligament. Along its course the internal saphenous vein receives many cutaneous branches from the leg and thigh and at the saphenous opening receives the superficial epigastric, superficial circumflex and the external pudic veins. The valves in this vein may number two to six and are usually more numerous in the thigh.

2. The external or short saphenous vein arises at the lateral side of the dorsum of the foot, ascends posteriorly to the external malleolus crossing the tendo Achilles to the midline of the posterior surface of the leg. From here it passes upward to terminate deeply in the popliteal vein. It contains from nine to twelve valves one of which is always found near its entrance into the popliteal vein.

B. Deep Veins of the Lower Extremities.

1. These accompany the arteries and their branches. All deep veins of the lower extremities contain numerous valves. They consist of:

a. The deep veins of the foot.

b. Anterior and posterior tibial veins.

c. The popliteal vein.

d. Femoral vein.

e. Deep femoral vein.

[3]

Lymphatics of the Lower Extremities

A. Lymphatic Vessels of the Lower Extremities.
   1. These consist of superficial and deep sets which follow the distribution of the veins very closely.
B. The Lymph Nodes.
   1. The anterior tibial node.
   2. The popliteal nodes embodied in the popliteal space.
   3. The inguinal nodes which are divided into:
      a. Superficial.
      b. Deep.

Veins of the Upper Extremities

A. Superficial Veins.
   1. Dorsal digital veins.
   2. Dorsal interosseous veins.
   3. Palmar plexus.
   4. Anterior ulnar vein.
      a. Ascends along the anterior surface of the ulnar side of the forearm to the elbow where it meets the posterior ulnar vein to form the common ulnar.
   5. Posterior ulnar vein.
      a. Runs along the posterior surface of the ulnar side of the forearm to just below the elbow where it joins the anterior ulnar vein to form the common ulnar.
   6. Common ulnar vein.
      a. When present, passes upward and laterally to join the median basilic vein and thus forms the basilic vein.
      b. May be absent, in which case the anterior and posterior ulnar veins empty separately into the medial basilic.
   7. Radial vein.
      a. Runs along the radial side of the forearm to the elbow region where it joins the median cephalic vein to form the cephalic.
   8. The median vein courses along the front of the forearm to the elbow region where it divides into median cephalic and median basilic veins.

[4]

    a. The median cephalic passes along the groove between the brachioradialis and biceps muscles, and together with the radial, forms the cephalic vein.

    b. The median basilic passes along the groove between the biceps and pronator teres muscles, and with the common ulnar, forms the basilic vein.

9. The basilic vein is formed by the junction of the common ulnar and the median basilic, passes up along the medial border of the biceps muscle to the middle of the arm where it goes through the deep fascia and travels with the brachial artery to the lower border of the latissimus dorsi and teres major tendons, where it becomes the axillary vein.

10. The cephalic vein comprises the union of the medial cephalic and radial veins. It travels along the lateral border of the biceps to the upper third of the arm where it pierces the costocoracoid membrane and ends as the axillary vein just below the clavicle.

11. The accessory cephalic vein runs along the back of the forearm to join the cephalic just above the elbow.

B. Deep Veins.

1. Follow the course of the arteries.

2. Usually one vein lying on each side of the artery, connected at intervals by short transverse branches.

3. The main deep veins are:

    a. Digital.

    b. Interosseous.

    c. Deep palmar.

    d. Brachial.

    e. Axillary.

        (1) This vein is the continuation of the basilic. It starts at the lower border of teres major tendon and stops beneath the clavicle at the outer border of the first rib, where it becomes the subclavian vein. Its branches are:

            (a) Long thoracic.

            (b) Thoracico-epigastric.

            (c) Costo-axillary.

    f. Subclavian.

        (1) This is a continuation of the axillary, extending from the lateral border of the first rib to the medial end of

the clavicle, where it joins the internal jugular to form the innominate vein.

Lymphatics of the Upper Extremities

A. Lymph Nodes.
  1. Antecubital.
      a. In front of the elbow.
  2. Epitrochlear.
      a. One or two nodes above the internal condyle.
  3. Infraclavicular.
      a. In groove between deltoid and pectoralis major muscles.
  4. Axillary.
      a. Drain the upper extremity, skin of upper thorax, pectoralis muscles and mammary gland.
B. Lymphatic Vessels.
  1. Superficial.
      a. Begin in the skin and ascend in subcutaneous tissues, terminating in superficial and deep nodes.
  2. Deep.
      a. Pass up the limb with the main vessels, draining the bone, periosteum, muscle and ligaments, terminating in the axillary nodes.

Arteries of the Upper Extremities

A. The Subclavian Arteries.
  1. The right subclavian artery takes origin from the innominate artery opposite the right sterno-clavicular articulation.
      a. It passes up and medially to the medial border of the scalenus anticus muscle, just above the clavicle.
      b. Continues behind the scalenus anticus muscle, then down and laterally to the lateral border of the first rib where it becomes the axillary artery.
  2. The left subclavian artery arises from the arch of the aorta, behind the left common carotid, ascends vertically and then arches laterally to the medial border of the scalenus anticus muscle.

[6]

    a. It continues behind the scalenus anticus muscle, then down and laterally to the first rib where it becomes the axillary artery.

3. The branches of the subclavian artery are:

    a. The vertebral.

    b. The thyroid axis.

        (1) Inferior thyroid.

        (2) Suprascapular.

        (3) Transverse cervical.

    c. Internal mammary.

    d. Superior intercostal.

B. The Axillary Artery.

1. This is a continuation of the subclavian. It commences at the outer margin of the first rib and ends at the lower border of the teres major tendon, where it becomes the brachial artery.

2. The branches of the axillary are:

    a. Superior thoracic.

    b. Acromiothoracic.

    c. Long thoracic.

    d. Alar thoracic.

    e. Subscapular.

    f. Posterior circumflex.

    g. Anterior circumflex.

C. The Brachial Artery.

1. This is a continuation of the axillary artery, passes down the medial and anterior aspect of the arm to just below the bend of the elbow where it divides into the radial and ulnar arteries.

2. The branches of the brachial artery are:

    a. Superior profunda.

    b. Inferior profunda.

    c. Nutrient.

    d. Anastomotica magna.

    e. Muscular.

D. The Radial Artery.

1. This commences at the bifurcation of the brachial and passes along the radial side of the forearm to the wrist; then turns behind the lateral margin of the carpus to the upper end of the space between the metacarpals of the thumb and index finger—

then passes into the palm of the hand, where it crosses the metacarpals to form the deep palmar arch.

2. The branches of the radial artery are:
   a. Radial recurrent.
   b. Muscular.
   c. Anterior radial carpal.
   d. Superficialis volae.
   e. Posterior radial carpal.
   f. First dorsal interosseous.
   g. Dorsalis pollicis.
   h. Dorsalis indicis.
   i. Princeps pollicis.
   j. Radialis indicis.
   k. Perforating.
   l. Palmar interosseous.
   m. Palmar recurrent.

E. The Ulnar Artery.

1. Starts just below the bend of the elbow, passes across the medial side of the forearm and then runs along the ulnar border to the wrist, crosses the annular ligament and just beyond the pisiform bone enters into the superficial and deep palmar arches.
2. The branches of the ulnar artery are:
   a. Anterior ulnar recurrent.
   b. Posterior ulnar recurrent.
   c. Interosseous.
   d. Muscular.
   e. Anterior ulnar carpal.
   f. Posterior ulnar carpal.
   g. Profunda.
   h. Superficial palmar arch.

F. The Superficial Palmar Arch.

1. This is formed by the ulnar artery in the hand and receives a branch from the radialis indicis, but sometimes by the superficialis volae or the princeps pollicis.
2. The branches of the superficial palmar arch are:
   a. Four digital arteries.

BIBLIOGRAPHY

Bardeleben, K., and Haeckel, H.: *Atlas of Applied* (*Topographical*) *Human Anatomy,* Rebman Co., 1906.

Gray's Anatomy: Lea & Febiger.

Lake, N. C.: *The Foot,* Wm. Wood & Co., 1935.

Lewin, P.: *The Foot and Ankle,* Lea & Febiger, 1940.

Vaus, P. N.: *The Anatomy of the Leg and Foot,* Wm. Wood & Co., 1935.

II

ANATOMY OF THE AUTONOMIC NERVOUS SYSTEM

A. Nomenclature.
   1. The autonomic nervous system is also sometimes called the involuntary or vegetative nervous system. It includes:
      a. The craniosacral or parasympathetic division which is derived from:
         (1) The 3rd, 7th, 9th, and 10th cranial nerves.
         (2) The 2nd, 3rd, and 4th sacral nerves.
      b. The thoracolumbar or sympathetic division which is derived from:
         (1) 1st to 12th thoracic nerves.
         (2) 1st and 2nd lumbar nerves.

B. Cranial Autonomic Centers.
   1. These are located in:
      a. The cerebral cortex.
         (1) These have not been definitely localized but probably do exist.
      b. The diencephalon.
         (1) These control visceral functions and probably some of the emotions.
      c. The medulla.
         (1) These affect the pupil, salivary glands and probably the heart and gastro-intestinal system.

C. The Thoracolumbar Division.
   1. This consists of:
      a. Spinal cord sympathetic channels in:
         (1) The anterior columns.
         (2) The pyramidal tracts.
         (3) The intermediolateral column.
         (4) The anterolateral spinothalamic tracts.
      b. The paravertebral sympathetic ganglia with rami communicantes. These are:

(1) The superior cervical ganglion which is opposite the 2nd and 3rd cervical vertebra.

(2) The middle cervical ganglion, which may be absent, lies at the level of the 6th cervical vertebra behind or in front of the inferior thyroid artery.

(3) The inferior cervical ganglion, usually fused with the 1st thoracic ganglion is known as the cervicothoracic or stellate ganglion. This lies between the head of the 1st rib and the vertebral artery where it joins the subclavian.

(4) The thoracic, lumbar and sacral ganglia show frequent variations in size and position.

    (a) They connect the spinal cord with the smooth muscle and glands of the body.

D. The Sympathetic Ganglia.

1. Connect centrally with the spinal nerves by means of white rami communicantes.

    a. These rami carry the preganglionic neurones.

        (1) There are no white rami in the cervical, lower lumbar or sacral segments.

2. Connect peripherally, to outlying organs by means of the gray rami communicantes.

E. Nerve Supply of the Peripheral Arteries.

This is received from:

1. The parasympathetic system.

    a. By means of vasodilation fibres which leave the spinal cord over the posterior roots.

2. The sympathetic system.

    a. By means of preganglionic neurones coming throughout the thoracolumbar portion of the intermediolateral column.

    b. These neurones emerge over the anterior roots and the white rami communicantes, ending in the ganglia of the paravertebral sympathetic chains.

        (1) Postganglionic neurones leave the paravertebral sympathetic ganglia and lead to:

            (a) The aorta, carotid, subclavian and iliac vessels.

            (b) All the arteries of the trunk and extremities by means of gray rami which lead back into the cervical, intercostal and lower spinal nerves.

BIBLIOGRAPHY

Gask, G. E., and Ross, J. P.: *The Surgery of the Sympathetic Nervous System*, Wm. Wood & Co., 1934.

White, J. C.: *The Autonomic Nervous System*, The Macmillan Co., 1935.

III

CLASSIFICATION OF PERIPHERAL VASCULAR DISEASES

A. The Organic Diseases.
  1. Arteriosclerosis.
  a. This may be present as a pathologic change in the arterial walls without narrowing the lumen or without causing obstruction by thrombi or ulceration. This type causes no clinical symptoms or objective signs.
    (1) The arteries may show calcification on roentgen examination without signs or symptoms of obstruction.
  b. It may be associated with hypertension and other visceral manifestations of arteriosclerosis but not necessarily.
  c. May be present as arteriolosclerosis, with renal, cardiac, cerebral, or peripheral vascular lesions.
  2. Arteriosclerosis obliterans.
  a. This is the same as arteriosclerosis with the addition of obstruction to blood flow caused by either narrowing of the arterial lumen or blockage by a thrombus.
  b. This gives rise to subjective and objective signs.
    (1) Objective signs may be present without any symptoms.
    (2) Symptoms may be out of all proportion to the objective findings.
  c. This process is probably accelerated by long-continued, neglected diabetes.
  d. Calcification of the arteries may or may not be visible on roentgen examination.
  3. Thrombo-angiitis obliterans (Buerger's disease).
  a. An inflammatory, undoubtedly infectious disease involving the arteries and veins of the extremities and occasionally the visceral arteries.
  4. Embolism of the peripheral arteries.
  5. Aneurysm of the peripheral arteries.

[13]

    a. Usually traumatic, especially when present as abnormal arteriovenous communication.

    b. May be congenital.

6. Tuberculosis and syphilis of the peripheral arteries.

    a. Extremely rare.

7. Periarteritis nodosa.

    a. Usually a generalized disease.

8. Subclavian artery obstruction.

    a. Due to either cervical rib or fibrotic scalenus anticus muscle.

9. Frost-bite.

10. Ergotism.

11. Glomus tumor.

B. The Functional Diseases.

    1. Raynaud's disease.

    2. Erythromelalgia.

    3. Acrocyanosis.

IV

SYMPTOMATOLOGY OF PERIPHERAL ARTERIAL DISEASES

A. Symptoms.

These may vary considerably and may include any or all of the following. These symptoms, as a rule, are initiated or aggravated by walking.

1. Burning sensation in various parts of the foot.
    a. Usually intensified by walking.
    b. May be worse at night.
    c. May be caused by tinea infections in the interdigital spaces.
2. Pain in the toes, foot or leg.
    a. Not felt while at rest.
    b. Usually in calf after walking.
    c. May resemble sciatica.
    d. May indicate impending gangrene.
    e. In embolism, is sudden in onset and may invade the entire leg.
3. Numbness of the toes or foot.
    a. Most pronounced in diabetic patients.
    b. May be accompanied by anesthesia of the foot.
    c. An early sign in arteriosclerosis obliterans.
    d. May indicate a spinal cord disease.
4. Intermittent claudication which may express itself as:
    a. Tired feeling in calf or leg.
        (1) Brought on by walking.
        (2) Worse on city pavements—not felt indoors as a rule.
        (3) Compels patient to stop and rest for a while.
        (4) Not present in Raynaud's disease.
        (5) May be the earliest sign of peripheral arterial disease.
        (6) Occurs in arms also, particularly in advanced thrombo-angiitis obliterans.
        (7) Is influenced a great deal by psychic factors, hence

should not be used as an indication of clinical improvement.

b. Cramp-like sensation.

    (1) In advanced cases, causing patient to stop walking.

c. Sharp pain in the calf.

    (1) Not present in Raynaud's disease.

    (2) Very severe and sudden in onset in embolism and thrombosis of large vessels of the extremities.

    (3) Must be differentiated from the sudden pain of ruptured plantaris muscle, a common occurrence, accompanied by hemorrhage between the soleus and gastrocnemius muscles, with ecchymosis of the leg and ankle.

d. Pain in the buttock radiating down the thigh.

    (1) Often confused with sciatica, which can be ruled out by negative Laségue's sign.

5. Rest pain occurs in advanced stages and is not influenced by exertion.

    a. Usually indicates impending gangrene.

    b. Worse in toes and foot.

    c. Not present in Raynaud syndrome.

    d. Intensified by smoking.

    e. Very severe in some stages of thrombo-angiitis obliterans.

    f. May cause patient to walk about room at night.

    g. Not controlled by nerve block.

    h. A diffuse tissue pain.

    i. May have associated neuritis.

    j. May be present in embolism of extremities.

6. Coldness of the feet.

    a. An early sign of all arterial diseases of the extremities.

    b. May indicate thrombosis or embolism.

    c. Usually present in Raynaud's disease.

    d. May indicate impending gangrene.

    e. May involve entire extremity.

7. Cessation of perspiration of affected foot.

    a. An early sign in thrombo-angiitis obliterans, first described by author.

    b. May be due to disturbance of sympathetic nervous system, common in early stages of thrombo-angiitis obliterans.

BIBLIOGRAPHY

Craig, W. M., and Ghormley, R. K.: 'Significance and Treatment of Sciatic Pain,' *J. A. M. A.*, 1933-100-1143.
Libman, E.: 'Observations of Individual Sensitiveness to Pain,' *J. A. M. A.*, 1934-102-335.

V

OBJECTIVE SIGNS OF ARTERIAL OCCLUSION

A. **Atrophy of Calf Muscles.**
   1. An early sign in organic disease.
   2. More evident as the disease progresses.
   3. May be due to poor nutrition of muscles or to disease.
B. **Nutritional Skin Disturbances of Extremities.**
   1. Atrophy and deformity of nails is usually due to fungus infection.
   2. Skin is shiny.
   3. Lanugo disappears.
C. **Disturbed Hair Growth of Extremities.**
   1. Lanugo becomes less, particularly on toes.
D. **Poorly Nourished and Deformed Toenails.**
   1. Usually due to fungus infection, particularly in diabetes.
   2. Nails may show transverse ridges.
   3. Usually dry, brittle and discolored.
E. **Relative Loss of Perspiration of Affected Limb.**
   1. Undoubtedly a disturbance of sympathetic nervous system, particularly in early stages of thrombo-angiitis obliterans.
F. **Plantar and Palmar Ischemia.**
   1. This is demonstrated by Samuels' test which is performed as follows:
      a. Feet are elevated to an angle of about 45° and while in this position flexion and extension of the ankle joints is carried out for a few minutes. Plantar ischemia will develop in direct proportion to the extent of arterial occlusion in the extremity. This sign is pathognomonic of organic arterial obstruction.
      b. For the upper extremities both hands are held above the head with the palms facing the observer. The hands are alternately opened and closed and finally maintained in the open position. Ischemia of fingers or palms denotes arterial obstruction. This test is often positive in advanced thrombo-

angiitis obliterans where involvement of the upper extremities is common.

G. Allen Test.

1. This is for the determination of patency of the ulnar artery only and is performed as follows:
   a. The hand is held above the head until blanching appears.
   b. The examiner then compresses the patient's radial artery and while maintaining the pressure brings the patient's hand down and observes the resulting color. Persistence of blanching in the dependent position indicates closure of the ulnar artery. Return of color indicates patency of the vessel.

H. Rubor.

1. Indicates long standing arterial disease.
2. It is not present in early cases.
3. Not present in Raynaud's disease.
4. Is not a diagnostic sign.
5. Also known as erythromelia.
6. It is characteristic of the disease erythromelalgia, especially when accompanied by burning sensation in the feet.
7. May occur in either thrombo-angiitis obliterans or arteriosclerosis obliterans.
8. May extend up to the knee.

I. Cyanosis of the Extremities.

1. In organic disease indicates impending gangrene. In vasomotor disturbances it is transient and not of serious consequence.
2. If cyanosis persists after pressure by the examining finger, gangrene is imminent.
3. If accompanied by coldness and severe pain, a sure sign of gangrene.
4. When present in Raynaud's disease it is usually followed by redness and is preceded by blanching of the parts.

J. Objective Coldness of Extremities.

1. May be determined by palpation with the palm or back of the hand.
   a. Comparison of each extremity is essential.
   b. Objective coldness may be present with absence of subjective coldness.

c. Extreme coldness plus cyanosis indicate impending gangrene.

d. Coldness of individual digits indicates digital artery obstruction.

2. By the use of an electrical thermometer such as the Dermalor or thermocouple.

a. For accurate results these apparatuses require a constant temperature room for the examination.

b. These instruments are particularly valuable in research and experimental work but are not necessary for routine clinical examinations.

c. The Dermalor, operating on the principle of the Wheatstone Bridge, is the simplest to operate and read.

(1) Mere contact of the wire electrode with the skin gives a direct reading in either centigrade or Fahrenheit.

d. Other apparatuses are available for deep muscle temperature determinations and for recording changes in skin and muscle temperature.

K. Palpation of Peripheral Arteries.

1. The dorsalis pedis artery may be congenitally absent.
2. The dorsalis pedis artery may be misplaced.
3. Edema may mask the pulsation of the artery.
4. The examiner may feel the pulse of his own fingers and mistake it for the patient's artery.
5. Arteries normally accessible to palpation are:

a. Dorsalis pedis.
b. Posterior tibial.
c. Anterior tibial.
d. Popliteal.
e. Femoral.
f. External iliac.
g. Axillary.
h. Brachial.
i. Radial.
j. Ulnar.

L. Histamine Test.

1. This indicates the status of the superficial circulation of the extremities and is not very reliable. It is performed as follows:

a. After thoroughly cleansing the skin of the area to be examined a drop of histamine phosphate is applied to the skin and a few scratch marks are made through the drop. After a few minutes a flare with a central area surrounded by a purpuric spot and a halo of rubor should appear. If the circulation is defective the flare either does not appear or is delayed.

M. Intracutaneous Salt Solution Test.

1. This is another unreliable procedure for determining the status of the circulation in the extremities. The test is carried out as follows:

a. 0.2 cc. of normal sodium chloride solution is injected at various levels of the leg and thigh into the skin. The wheals thus formed should disappear in about an hour if the circulation is normal.

N. Arteriography.

1. Roentgen visualization of the arteries of the living extremity should be employed only in the diagnosis of unusual conditions such as arteriovenous aneurysm. Any of the following substances may be used: diodrast, neoskiodan or thorotrast. The technic of arteriography is as follows:

a. In the upper extremity a blood pressure cuff is applied high up in the axilla.

b. The skin and subcutaneous tissues are injected with novocain just above the lacertus fibrosus. At this point the brachial artery is punctured with an ordinary intravenous needle and the opaque material is injected. One ampoule of solution is usually sufficient.

c. As soon as the brachial artery has been punctured the blood pressure cuff is inflated to prevent spread of the fluid. A roentgen exposure is made immediately after withdrawal of the needle with subsequent exposures as necessary. In the lower extremity the femoral artery is punctured in the same manner just below Poupart's ligament. Instead of a blood pressure cuff the artery may be compressed by an assistant.

O. Capillary Studies.

1. These are interesting but have so far afforded no trustworthy diagnostic information.

P. Oscillometry.
1. For accurate quantitative measurement of arterial pulsation an oscillometer is indispensable.
    a. Types of oscillometers.
        (1) Pachon.
            (a) Obsolete but very efficient.
        (2) Boulitte.
            (a) Excellent but complicated in operation.
        (3) Hellige-Samuels pulsimeter.
            (a) Simplest to operate.
            (b) Inexpensive.
        (4) Tycos recording.
            (a) Furnishes tracings of pulses.
            (b) Expensive.
            (c) Indispensable for research.
    b. Normal readings fall within a wide range but should be somewhat as follows:
        (1) Axillary region, 4 to 20.
        (2) Brachial, 2 to 12.
        (3) Wrist, 1 to 10.
        (4) Palm, 0.5 to 2.
        (5) Upper thigh, 4 to 16.
        (6) Lower thigh, 4 to 14.
        (7) Calf, 3 to 10.
        (8) Ankle, 1 to 10.
        (9) Foot, 0.5 to 4.
    c. A zero reading at the ankle indicates closure of main arterial channels with consequent poor collateral circulation indicating grave prognosis.

BIBLIOGRAPHY

Allen, E. V.: 'Thrombo-angiitis Obliterans: Methods of Diagnosis of Chronic Occlusive Arterial Lesions Distal to the Wrist with Illustrative Cases,' *Am. J. M. Sc.,* 1929-178-237.

Allen, E. V., and Camp, J. D.: 'Arteriography, a Roentgenographic Study of the Peripheral Arteries of the Living Subject Following Their Injection with a Radiopaque Substance,' *J. A. M. A.,* 1935-104-618.

BIBLIOGRAPHY

Atlas, L. N.: 'Oscillometric Readings in Cases of Arteriosclerotic Disease of Lower Extremity, Significance and Interpretation,' *Arch. Int. M.,* 1940-66-155.

'Oscillometry in Diagnosis of Arteriosclerosis of Lower Extremties: New Method of Application,' *Arch. Int. M.,* 1939-63-1158.

Baggenstass, A. H., and Keith, H. N.: 'Calcification of the Arteries of an Infant,' *Proc. Staff Meet., Mayo Clin.,* 1941-16-120.

Berberich, J., and Hirsch, S.: 'Die röntgenographische Darstellung der Arterien und Venen am lebenden Menschen,' *Klin. Wchnschr.,* Berl., 1923-2-2226.

Berk, J. E.: 'Circulation Time (Magnesium Sulfate Method) in Diagnosis of Peripheral Vascular Disease,' *Am. J. M. Sc.,* 1940-199-505.

Bloom, N.: 'Tests for Peripheral Circulatory Efficiency,' *Virginia M. Monthly,* 1939-66-478.

Brooks, B.: 'Intra-arterial Injection of Sodium Iodide,' *J. A. M. A.,* 1924-82-1016.

Determann, H.: 'Intermittierendes Hinken eines Arms, der Zunge und der Beine (Dyskinesia Intermittens Angio-Sclerotica),' *Deutsch. Ztschr. F. Nervenh.,* 1905-29-152.

Dos-Santos, R., Lamas, A. C., and Caldas, J. P.: *Artériographie des membres et de l'aorte abdominale,* Masson et Cie, Paris, 1931.

Duryee, A. W., and Wright, I. S.: 'Studies of Human Capillaries,' *Am. J. M. Sc.,* 1933-185-664.

Kvale, W. F., and Allen, E. V.: 'The Rate of Circulation in the Arteries and Veins of Man. I. Studies of Normal Subjects and of Those with Occlusive Arterial Disease and Hyperthyroidism,' *Am. Heart J.,* 1939-18-519.

'The rate of the Circulation in the Arteries and Veins of Man. III. The Influence of Temperature of the Skin, Digestion, Posture, and Exercise,' *Am. Heart J.,* 1939-18-546.

'The Rate of the Circulation in the Arteries and Veins of Man. IV. An Error in the Sodium Cyanide Method of Determining Speed of Venous Blood Flow,' *Am. Heart J.,* 1939-18-557.

Kvale, W. F., Allen, E. V., and Adson, A. W.: 'The Rate of the Circulation in the Arteries and Veins of Man. II. Studies of Hypertension, of Orthostatic Hypotension, and of the Effects of Sympathectomy,' *Am. Heart J.,* 1939-18-537.

Lange, K., and Boyd, L. J.: 'Use of Fluorescein Method in Establishment of Diagnosis and Prognosis of Peripheral Vascular Diseases,' *Arch. Int. Med.*, 1944-74-175.

Laveran, A.: 'Observation d'endarterite oblitérante avec gangrène des extrémités inférieures,' *Bull. de l'Academie de Med.*, 1894-31-191.

Lewis, T.: *Blood Vessels of the Human Skin and Their Responses*, Shaw and Sons, London, 1927.

McClure, W. B., and Aldrich, C. A.: 'Time Required for Disappearance of Intradermal Injected Salt Solution,' *J. A. M. A.*, 1923-81-293.

Moffat, D. A.: 'The Modern Apparatus and Technic for the Study of Diseases of the Peripheral Vascular System,' *M. Clin. North America*, 1934-17-92.

Morton, J. J., and Scott, W. J. M.: 'The Measurement of Sympathetic Vasoconstriction Activity in the Lower Extremities,' *J. Clin. Invest.*, 1930-9-235.

Oehler, J.: 'Über einen bemerkenswerten Fall von Dyskinesia intermittens Brachiorum,' *Deutsch. Arch. f. klin. Med.*, 1907-08-92-154.

Redisch, W.: 'Zur Kapillarmikroskopie und Kapillarphotographie,' *Zeitschr. f. Kreislaufforschung*, 1930-22-561.

Samuels, S. S.: 'The Early Diagnosis of Thrombo-angiitis Obliterans: a new diagnostic sign,' *J. A. M. A.*, 1929-92-1571.

'Peripheral Arterial Diseases—The Fundamentals in Their Diagnosis and Treatment,' *J. M. Soc. New Jersey*, 1938-35-224.

Wagner, F. B.: 'Complications Following Arteriography of Peripheral Vessels,' *J. A. M. A.*, 1944-125-958.

Weber, F. P.: 'Arteritis Obliterans of the Lower Extremities with Intermittent Claudication,' *Proc. Roy. Soc. Med.*, 1907-1-44.

VI

ARTERIOSCLEROSIS OBLITERANS

A. Etiology.
  1. Age.
    a. Arteriosclerosis occurs most often after age thirty, although cases have been observed in younger individuals, particularly in combination with diabetes mellitus.
  2. Heredity.
    a. The family incidence is very high and there seems to be a hereditary tendency.
  3. Theory of Winternitz, Thomas and LeCompte.
    a. Arteriosclerosis is a tissue reaction to unknown toxic or bacterial agents.
  4. Sex.
    a. It is more prevalent in men although not to the same degree as thrombo-angiitis obliterans.
  5. It is apparently influenced by uncontrolled diabetes and polycythemia, each of which seems to intensify the arteriosclerotic process.
B. Pathology.
  1. The intimal type of arteriosclerosis is most common in peripheral arterial diseases. When accompanied by clinical evidence of obstruction to arterial onflow it is known as arteriosclerosis obliterans.
    a. The intima is thickened. The media shows new connective tissue and wandering cells loaded with fat.
    b. The fatty areas may become necrotic and thrombi may form.
    c. The necrotic areas may become calcified and be visible on roentgen examination.
      (1) Obstructing thrombi may form suddenly on calcified plaques, producing a clinical picture strongly resembling embolism. Differentiation between these conditions is often difficult.

2. The Mönckeberg type of arteriosclerosis is usually confined to the femoral arteries with very little change in the intima; usually calcification of the media which does not cause obstruction because the vessels become dilated instead of obstructed.

3. Associated arteriosclerotic manifestations.

    a. The coronary arteries are often involved as well as vessels of the brain, spinal cord and retina.

    b. The abdominal and pulmonary arteries are rarely involved.

C. Symptoms.

    1. Paresthesias of the toes and feet are common.

        a. May be present in early stages.

        b. May be the only symptom.

    2. Pain in buttock resembling sciatica.

        a. Usually radiates down the back of the leg.

        b. May be present in all stages.

    3. Subjective coldness of feet.

        a. An important symptom, particularly in sudden thrombosis of large arteries.

    4. Intermittent claudication.

        a. A tired feeling, cramp or pain in the calf of the affected leg on walking.

            (1) Not noticeable indoors, but always on walking outdoors.

            (2) In advanced cases the patient may be able to walk only one block or less.

            (3) Some patients, with diminished pain sensibility may walk long distances in spite of extensive arterial disease.

            (4) This symptom is frequently influenced by psychic factors, hence it cannot be used as a gauge of clinical improvement.

    5. Rest pain is usually constant day and night and may signify impending gangrene.

        a. Not present in early cases.

        b. May be associated with diabetic neuritis.

D. Objective Findings.

    1. Samuels' test for plantar ischemia is always positive in organic arterial obstruction in the extremities.

        a. This test is carried out by having the patient lie with the feet elevated at an angle of about 45°.

   b. Rapid flexing and extension of the ankle joints is now carried out for a minute or two and the soles of the feet are examined in a good, even light. Plantar pallor indicates arterial obstruction, usually in direct proportion to the amount of obstruction present.

2. Relative coldness of the involved foot is fairly constant.

   a. This may be determined either by palpation or by an electrical apparatus.

   b. The pale foot is usually cold.

3. Rubor is present in advanced cases only.

   a. It has limited diagnostic value.

4. Cyanosis denotes either long-standing obstruction or impending gangrene, usually the latter.

   a. If it disappears after pressure with the examining finger, the significance of it is not too serious.

5. Edema of the feet and legs may be due to a local condition or cardiorenal insufficiency.

   a. As a rule it indicates maintenance of the legs in the dependent position. This is bad and may be overcome by changing to the horizontal position.

   b. Edema hinders healing of ulcers and gangrene.

6. Relative atrophy of the calf muscles of the affected leg is a frequent finding.

   a. It is usually associated with the conditions described above.

7. Tinea infections may be present in plantar calluses, interdigital fissures or around base of toenails.

   a. They are a frequent source of infection and gangrene, particularly in diabetes.

8. The palpability of the dorsalis pedis and posterior tibial pulses is not essential for diagnosis as many cases of arteriosclerosis obliterans have palpable pulses with plantar ischemia and coldness.

   a. These pulses are frequently misplaced or otherwise difficult to palpate.

9. Oscillometry is an important part of the physical examination in diagnosis and prognosis.

   a. Opposite extremities should always be examined for comparative readings.

b. A zero reading at the ankle level indicates uncertain prognosis.

E. Treatment of Arteriosclerosis Obliterans.
  1. For ambulatory patients.
    a. Smoking must be strictly forbidden.
      (1) The vasoconstricting action of smoking is detrimental, especially in the early stages.
    b. Preservation of the natural warmth of the extremities is attained by the use of woolen socks and underwear.
      (1) External heat in the form of baking lamps, heating pads, hot water bottles and thermostatic cradles should not be used as severe burns may result.
        (a) Many cases of gangrene have been initiated by heating apparatuses.
    c. A daily hot sitz bath for ten-minute periods.
      (1) Temperature of the water should not be over 105° F.
      (2) The level of the water should be to the hips only.
      (3) Following the bath, the feet should be carefully dried and olive oil or lanolin applied.
    d. Short wave diathermy, three times a week for twenty-minute periods may be used in conjunction with other measures.
      (1) Should not be used in the presence of open lesions of the extremities.
      (2) The patient should control the current intensity personally to avoid overheating.
    e. Postural exercises. These consist of cycles of elevation, dependency and horizontal position of the legs carried out twice a day or oftener if possible.
      (1) The legs are elevated for two minutes, dependent for three minutes, horizontal two minutes. This is repeated four or five times in succession.
      (2) The exercises should not be done in the presence of acute inflammation.
      (3) They are most effective when followed immediately by the hot sitz bath.
    f. Intravenous injections of 2% sodium chloride solution 300 cc., three times a week for stimulation of the collateral cir-

culation may be used effectively in some cases in conjunction with other measures.

    (1) Contraindications are hypertension, cardiac disease, renal disease.

    (2) This is an office procedure and should have no unpleasant reaction.

g. For relief of rest pain or intermittent claudication, intramuscular injections of cobra venom or de-insulinized pancreatic extracts may be used.

    (1) Cobra venom is given intramuscularly in doses of 1 cc.—daily or oftener, if indicated.

        (a) No contraindications or reactions have been noted.

    (2) De-insulinized pancreatic extracts have no demonstrable effect upon the circulation.

        (a) Their value, if any, is in the relief of pain of intermittent claudication.

        (b) They have no effect upon rest pain.

        (c) They have no influence in the healing of ulcers or gangrene.

h. The following should be avoided in the treatment of arteriosclerosis obliterans because of the danger of sudden thrombosis of main arteries.

    (1) Intravenous injections of typhoid vaccine.

        (a) These cause a decrease in the coagulation time during the chill phase of the reaction.

    (2) Intermittent venous compression machines.

        (a) These machines very often damage the femoral vein or artery because of the excessive pressure of the cuff.

        (b) Instances of sudden thrombosis of the femoral vein and artery have been observed as a result of the use of these machines.

        (c) Any relief of pain is psychic and may be obtained with simpler and safer measures.

        (d) Ulcers that have apparently been healed by this method are usually amenable to bed rest.

(3) Suction and pressure machines.

    (a) These machines commonly known as pavex and by other trade names have demonstrated their worthlessness after years of trial by competent observers.

    (b) The pressure of the constricting rubber thigh cuff may, as in the intermittent venous compression machines, seriously damage the large vessels of the thigh, resulting in sudden thrombosis and massive gangrene.

    (c) The psychic effect of these apparatuses is tremendous as far as relief of symptoms is concerned, but the same results can be obtained with simpler and safer procedures.

(4) Vasodilating drugs.

    (a) The various vasodilating drugs such as the nitrites, acetylcholine and its derivatives, have no noticeable effect in the organic arterial diseases of the extremities unless given intravenously which is inadvisable in humans.

    (b) Mecholyl iontophoresis has been tried but has proven valueless and may be dangerous because of the ease of burning the tissues during treatment.

    (c) Papaverine may be effective in doses up to 10 grains per day when given by mouth.

    (d) Estrogens may have some vasodilating action.

    (e) Alcohol by mouth may be used as an effective vasodilator but should be prescribed with care in the case of habitual drunkards. Diabetes mellitus does not seem to be a contraindication to the use of alcohol in moderate amounts.

(5) Operations on the sympathetic nervous system.

    (a) The amount of vasospasm present in arteriosclerosis obliterans is negligible, except in the very early stages.

    (b) In the incipient cases the vasomotor disturbance can be effectively relieved with the simple and safe measures outlined above.

    (c) In the advanced cases where vasospasm plays a

secondary part or is practically absent, sympathectomy is of no value and can be dangerous.

(6) Peripheral nerve block or lumbar block with alcohol or novocain injections is not effective in arteriosclerosis obliterans and may have disastrous side effects.

2. Treatment of arteriosclerotic gangrene.

a. Complete bed rest in the early stages is essential.

(1) This is particularly true of incipient gangrene since it is impossible to derive any therapeutic benefit in these cases unless the patient has complete bed rest.

(2) If gangrene has developed, bed rest with the extremities in the horizontal position is obligatory.

(3) Infection, if present, is also controlled much better with the extremities at rest.

b. Preservation of the natural warmth of the extremity by wrapping with cotton from the toes to the groin is a routine procedure.

(1) It is a good plan to wrap both extremities to secure the maximum effects.

c. Intravenous injections of 300 cc. 2% sodium chloride solution three times a week where there is no contraindication.

(1) This form of therapy should be used in conjunction with all other methods described.

d. Severe pain of impending or developing gangrene may be controlled with intramuscular injections of cobra venom.

(1) Cobra venom may be given three or four times during the day if necessary with no fear of overdose or of unpleasant reactions.

(2) Whiskey in doses of 1 ounce three times a day may be helpful in the control of pain.

e. Smoking is contraindicated in any stage of arteriosclerosis obliterans and particularly in the case of impending or developing gangrene.

(1) The vasoconstricting action of nicotine is tremendous and pain is markedly increased while gangrene tends to spread.

f. Primary, ischemic or so-called 'dry gangrene' due to arterial occlusion exclusively is allowed to demarcate spontaneously applying daily dressings of azochloramide in triacetin 1 : 500. After a line of demarcation is established the gangrenous portion should be dissected away carefully with the application of azochloramide or ointment dressings until the stump granulates and heals.

(1) A gangrenous toe should not be removed until it is completely and thoroughly demarcated and dehydrated.

(a) The separation should be carried out carefully along the line of demarcation avoiding injury to the living tissue.

(b) Particular attention must be paid to the flexor tendon of the toe, cutting it in such a way that the proximal end will not retract into the sheath and thus cause infection.

(c) Penicillin should be administered before and after amputation of a toe as a prophylactic measure.

(2) All dressings must be done daily with extreme care to avoid the introduction of infection.

g. Secondary or infected gangrene previously known as 'wet gangrene.' Secondary gangrene is defined as a gangrenous process developing as a result of infection in an extremity with deficient arterial circulation.

(1) Causes of secondary gangrene.

(a) Fungus infections. These organisms may be present in interdigital spaces, in plantar calluses or in 'corns' in various parts of the feet.

(b) There are various strains of fungi which have not yet been completely classified. It may be that certain of these strains are responsible for the severe infections encountered in diabetic gangrene as well as in the gangrene of thrombo-angiitis obliterans.

(c) The fungi thrive in dead epithelium which accounts for their universal presence in calluses, corns and other epithelial thickenings.

(d) The introduction of secondary pyogenic organisms in the areas of tinea infections may produce gross infection. The resulting localized edema and swelling around the infected area causes further interference with the arterial blood supply to that locality. This causes death of tissue and gangrene.

(e) Trauma to the feet such as cutting 'corns,' calluses and trimming so-called ingrown toenails may also introduce secondary infected gangrene. The simultaneous presence of diabetes mellitus intensifies the infection and lowers resistance. Diabetic gangrene is, properly speaking, diabetic arteriosclerotic gangrene.

(2) Treatment of diabetic gangrene (secondary or infected arteriosclerotic gangrene). Since secondary gangrene arises primarily from an infection it is logical to treat the condition by eliminating the infection. This is done by the ordinary surgical methods of incision, drainage and the use of antiseptic solutions. Incisions, however, must follow anatomical lines as in the treatment of hand infections.

(a) There are three classical routes of infection in the feet.

(b) Dorsal infections. These usually follow the extensor tendons of the toes and are usually superficial and do not as a rule extend farther than the ankle level. Longitudinal incisions along the entire course of the tendon involved are usually sufficient.

(c) Dorsal infections as a rule are accompanied by spreading patches of gangrene of the dorsum of the foot due to pressure of the underlying infection. In making the incision to drain the infection on the dorsum of the foot it is well to excise all gangrenous parts, at the same time packing the entire cavity with azochloramide gauze.

(d) Flexor tendon sheath infections of the sole of the foot are most serious, particularly those involving the tendon sheath of the flexor longus hallucis. Involvement of these tendon sheaths may be diagnosed by pressure along the course of the tendon noting whether or not pus exudes proximally from the gangrenous area. If pressure at a distance does produce pus at the point of gangrene a grooved director is inserted along the tract of the tendon sheath and the entire area laid wide open with either a straight scissors or a scalpel. Never use a local anesthetic such as ethyl chloride or novocain for this operation as either of these may produce gangrene. As a rule no anesthesia is needed but in exceptional cases a general anesthetic may be used.

(e) Another common path of infection is along the transverse fatty areolar tissue fascial space at the base of the toes (subdigital space), running from the base of the great toe to that of the fifth toe. When this becomes involved, as noted by expression of pus, a longitudinal incision under the guidance of a grooved director along the base of the toes will prove sufficient. After proper incision has been made and all pus pockets thoroughly evacuated the cavities should be irrigated with hydrogen peroxide or azochloramide in saline 1 : 3300 and the cavities then packed thoroughly and tightly with gauze saturated with azochloramide in triacetin 1 : 500.

3. Chemotherapy in diabetic gangrene.

   a. As soon as the diagnosis of infection in the diabetic foot has been made, cultures of the infected area should be taken if possible and the appropriate chemotherapeutic agent immediately administered.

      (1) The great majority of these infections are of the staphylococcus group.

   b. Penicillin should be administered intramuscularly at the first sign of infection either in doses of 20,000 units every three hours or if given slowly, in a slowly absorbable base, in doses of 200,000 units daily. In those cases where azochloramide does not seem to be beneficial, local wet dressings of penicillin solution in normal saline, 500 units per cc. may be tried.

   c. Tyrothricin or streptomycin may be used instead of penicillin.

   d. It must be remembered that these agents are of no value unless at the same time the infected area is properly incised.

4. Treatment of diabetes in diabetic gangrene.

    a. As long as there is undrained infection in the foot it will be impossible to control the blood sugar or the glycosuria with large doses of insulin. As soon as the infection is properly controlled, however, the insulin requirement will drop considerably.

        (1) Protamine insulin should not be used during the acute stages of diabetic gangrene as it is difficult to control the dosage during the daily twenty-four hour period. Ordinary insulin may be administered in these cases more safely and more accurately.

        (2) In older patients it is not necessary to have the urine completely sugar-free nor to reduce the blood sugar to a normal level. Such action may result in the onset of anginal attacks.

5. Gas bacillus infections in diabetic gangrene of the feet are rare and avoidable. They usually arise from contamination with blankets and from careless dressing of the gangrenous area.

    a. It must be distinguished from infection with gas-producing organisms which are relatively benign such as anaerobic streptococci, colon bacilli and other gas-producing organisms.

        (1) These are readily identified by culture and by the fact that the generalized symptoms are not as severe as in true Welch bacillis infection. These benign gas infections respond to the routine treatment outlined above.

    b. True Welch bacillus infections on the other hand may often prove fatal in spite of all treatment and require, in addition to large incisions of the leg and foot, the use of gas bacillus sera, roentgen therapy, and chemotherapeutic agents. The use of zinc peroxide locally is also recommended in these cases. Penicillin may be used.

6. Prognosis in diabetic gangrene.

    a. An oscillometric reading of 0.5 or more at the ankle level in a case of diabetic gangrene indicates adequate collateral circulation and a good chance for healing under conservative therapy.

    b. A reading of zero at the ankle level indicates poor collateral circulation and a proportionately poor prognosis.

F. Indications for Amputation in Arteriosclerotic and Diabetic Gangrene.

    1. Gangrene of the foot of such extent that the weight-bearing portion of the extremity is destroyed.

    2. Infection of the foot of such severity that it cannot be controlled by ordinary means.

    3. Surgical amputation of involved toes in diabetic gangrene should never be done as pathways of infection are thereby opened and ultimate loss of the leg may result.

    4. Below-knee amputations are indicated only when the circulation in the extremity as shown by an oscillometer is adequate. In other words, when the oscillometric index at the ankle level is 1.0 or more. As these cases as a rule can be controlled with conservative treatment it is evident that amputation below the knee is seldom indicated.

G. Preparation for Operation.

    1. Adequate and careful preoperative preparation of the skin is essential.

        a. Before application of iodine the operative field is thoroughly scrubbed in the operating room first with benzine, then with alcohol.

        b. Careful draping of the leg is also essential.

    2. Site of amputation.

        a. The supracondylar amputation in the lower third of the thigh is the best and simplest operation for diabetic and arteriosclerotic gangrene.

    3. Cyclopropane or nitrous oxide gas are the anesthesias of choice. Spinal anesthesia should be avoided because there may be an unavoidable tendency for the blood pressure to drop during the administration of the anesthetic which may initiate a sudden thrombosis of the large vessels of the extremities followed by massive gangrene.

    4. Refrigeration anesthesia is unnecessary and presents the danger of gas-bacillus infection of the stump.

H. Technic of Leg Amputation.

    1. A circular incision is made through the skin and soft parts at the upper level of the patella. This is carried around in one

sweep down to the fascia and a fresh scalpel is then used for further dissection.

2. All soft parts are now cut in one plane without undermining skin, down to the bone. All bleeding vessels are clamped as the operation proceeds. No tourniquet is used.

3. When the bone is reached the soft parts are retracted proximally for about two inches with a wet towel and the femur is sawed through at the uppermost level of the operative field after first incising the periosteum and scraping it distilly.

    a. The soft parts now fall together without any tension over the ends of the cut bone and approximation of muscles and fascia is secured with the use of sutures applied without tension. Fine silk may be used.

4. After careful approximation of all soft parts the skin is closed carefully with silk sutures leaving no dead spaces and inserting no drains of any kind. A simple bandage is applied over the stump and the operation is finished.

5. The practice of leaving amputation stumps wide open or of inserting drains is unnecessary, dangerous and the cause of the present high mortality in the hands of some operators.

    a. Regardless of the extent of infection in the foot the supracondylar operative field is not infected except in the rare cases of true gas bacillus infection.

    b. Inserting drains and leaving stumps open invite contamination and destructive infection of the stump. With careful technic the most extensively infected diabetic foot may be removed by a supracondylar amputation with no danger of infection of the stump if the wound is sewed tight without drainage.

I. Postoperative Care.

1. If there is no contraindication the patient is allowed in a wheel chair the day after the operation and every day thereafter.

2. The regular preoperative diet is resumed on the day following operation, and insulin given as necessary.

3. As a rule skin sutures may be removed on the fifth to the seventh day and the patient may be discharged from the hospital on the eighth to the tenth day.

4. The patient may be up and walking about on crutches on the third to fifth day if conditions permit.

5. Mortality from this operation 7.5%.

6. An artificial limb may be applied as soon as the stump is firmly healed; three weeks after the operation is the average time for the use of an artificial limb.

J. Infection of Stump.

1. If the stump should become infected after the operation or if the skin flap should become gangrenous, the path of the infection should be opened carefully and not too radically, and penicillin used systemically and locally.

2. If the skin edges of the flaps become gangrenous, the sutures should be removed and the involved area treated with penicillin.

3. After granulations appear dressings of azochloramide in triacetin 1 : 500 may be used.

BIBLIOGRAPHY

Caizzone, G.: 'Diabetic Gangrene,' *Rassegna internaz. di clin. e. terap.*, 1936-17-351.

Conway, H., and Meigager, S. C.: 'Infection and Gangrene in the Lower Extremities and Diabetes Mellitus,' *N. Y. State J. of Med.*, 1942-42-519.

Cowdry, E. V.: *Arteriosclerosis*, The Macmillan Co., 1933.

Donehue, F. M.: 'Surgical Aspects of Diabetic Gangrene,' *N. Y. State J. of Med.*, 1942-42-511.

Fisher, M. A., Duryee, A. W., and Wright, I. S.: 'Deproteinated Pancreatic Extract (Depropanex).' '1. Effect in Treatment of Intermitted Claudication Due to Arteriosclerosis Obliterans,' *Am. Heart J.*, 1939-18-425.

Gardberg, M.: 'Diabetic Infection and Gangrene,' *New Orleans M. & S. J.*, 1937-89-362.

Gustafson, E.: 'Medical Aspects of Diabetic Gangrene,' *N. Y. State J. of Med.*, 1942-42-512.

Halford, A. C. F.: 'Diabetic Gangrene,' *M. J. Australia*, 1936-2-121.

Hines, E. A., Jr.: 'Thrombo-arteriosclerosis Obliterans: a clinical study of 280 cases,' *Proc. Staff Meet., Mayo Clin.*, 1938-13-694.

Hines, E. A., Jr., and Barker, N. W.: 'Arteriosclerosis Obliterans: a clinical and pathologic study,' *Am. J. Med. Sc.*, 1940-200-717.

BIBLIOGRAPHY

Joslin, P. J.: *The Treatment of Diabetes Mellitus,* Lea & Febiger, 1937.

Kanavel, A.: *Infections of the Hand,* Lea & Febiger, 1939.

Kelley, H. T.: 'Diabetes: III. Significance of Dermatophytosis in Diabetes,' *Penn. Med. J.,* 1940-43-1416.

Kirz, E., 'Gas Gangrene after Amputation under Refrigeration Anesthesia: A Warning,' *Brit. M. J.,* 1944-2-662.

Lansbury, J., and Brown, G. E.: 'The Clinical Significance of Calcification of the Arteries of the Lower Extremities,' *Proc. Staff Meet., Mayo Clin.,* 1934-9-49.

Leoni Iparraguirre, C. A.: 'Endarteritis Obliterans of the Lower Extremities,' *Dia Medico,* 1940-12-597.

Lisa, J. R., Magidy, M., and Hart, J. F.: 'Peripheral Arteriosclerosis in the Diabetic and Nondiabetic,' *J. A. M. A.,* 1942-118-1353.

Lundsgaard, C., and Rud, E.: 'Studies on Arteriosclerosis in the Peripheral Arteries by Means of X-rays,' *Acta Med. Scandinav.,* 1928-26-558.

McGrath, E. J., and Hermann, L. G., 'Effect of Estrogens on Peripheral Vascular Disease,' *Ann. Surgery,* 1944-120-607.

McKittrick, L. S.: 'Chronic Obliterative Vascular Disease,' *J. A. M. A.,* 1939-113-1223.

'Diabetic Gangrene—Review of 972 Cases of Gangrene Associated with Diabetes Mellitus Treated at the New England Deaconess Hospital,' *Arch. Surg.,* 1940-40-35.

McKittrick, L. S., and Root, H. F.: *Diabetic Surgery,* Lea & Febiger, 1928.

Meleney, F. L.: 'Zinc Peroxide in Treatment of Micro-aerophilic and Anaerobic Infections,' *Ann. Surg.,* 1935-101-997.

'Further Laboratory and Clinical Experience in Treatment of Chronic Undermining Burrowing Ulcers with Zinc Peroxide,' *Surgery,* 1937-1-169.

Meleney, F. L., and Johnson, B.: 'The Prophylactic and Active Treatment of Surgical Infections with Zinc Peroxide,' *Surg. Gynec. & Obst.,* 1937-64-387.

Mohs, F. E., Sevringhaus, E. L., and Schmidt, E. R.: 'Conservative Amputation of Gangrenous Parts by Chemosurgery,' *Ann. Surg.,* 1941-114-161.

Murray, G.: 'Diabetic Infection and Gangrene,' *Can. M. Ass. J.,* 1939-41-246.

[39]

Ochsner, A., and DeBakey, M.: 'Peripheral Vascular Disease: Critical Survey of Its Conservative and Radical Treatment,' *Surg. Gynec. & Obst.*, 1940-70-1058.

Pearl, F. L., and Kandel, A.: 'Peripheral Vascular Status of One Hundred Unselected Patients with Diabetes,' *J. A. M. A.*, 1939-39-86.

Perlow, S., and Halpern, S. S.: 'Surgical Relief of Pain Due to Circulatory Disturbances of Feet. Report of a New Method,' *Am. J. Surg.*, 1939-45-104.

Pennoyer, G. P.: 'Diabetic Gangrene,' *N. Y. State J. Med.*, 1942-42-507.

Pratt, T. C.: 'General Management and Treatment of Peripheral Vascular Disease of Lower Extremities,' *New Eng. J. M.*, 1937-216-493.

Samuels, S. S.: 'Fundamental Principles in the Treatment of Diabetic Gangrene,' *Surgery*, 1937-2-225.

'Leg Amputations in Diabetic Gangrene,' *Ann. Surg.*, 1940-112-105.

'The Conservative Treatment of Diabetic Gangrene,' *Surg. Gynec. & Obst.*, 1939-69-342.

'Treatment of Diabetic Gangrene,' *Bull. Hosp. Joint Dis.*, 1943-4-16.

Solley, F. W.: 'Diabetic Lower Extremity Amputations,' *N. Y. State J. Med.*, 1942-42-507.

Warfield, J. O.: 'Diabetic Gangrene—Complicated by Welch Bacillus Infection,' *M. Ann. Dist. of Col.*, 1936-5-H207.

Weber, F. P.: 'Arteritis Obliterans of the Lower Extremities with Intermittent Claudication,' *Proc. Roy. Soc. Med.*, 1907-1-44.

Winternitz, M. C., Thomas, R. M., and LeCompte, P. M.: *The Biology of Arteriosclerosis*, Chas. C. Thomas, Springfield, 1938.

VII

THROMBO-ANGIITIS OBLITERANS

A. Etiology.

1. Unknown, although a low-grade infection seems the most likely cause. Possibility of a fungus infection of the feet with extension to the arteries and veins of the extremities must be considered as a cause of this disease. Tobacco, particularly smoking, is an aggravating factor as far as the circulation is concerned inasmuch as the vasoconstricting action is definitely harmful in any arterial disturbance of the extremities.

   a. Streptococcus and other bacteria have been suggested as possible causes, but experimental work so far has not been sufficiently conclusive to warrant the assumption.

   b. The role of fungi in the causation and spread of gangrene in thrombo-angiitis obliterans is undoubtedly of prime importance, from the clinical appearance of the lesions and their progress.

B. Race.

1. It may affect any member of the human race but is presumed to be more prevalent in the Russian Jew.

2. Cases have been seen in the following nationalities: Irish, Italians, Swedes, Norwegians, Chinese, Japanese, Germans.

3. Although many cases have been reported in Negroes, the evidence shown as proof of the diagnosis of thrombo-angiitis obliterans is not sufficiently convincing to establish this point.

C. Sex.

1. The disease is generally predominant in the male sex although occasional instances in females have been seen and reported.

   a. To establish the diagnosis of thrombo-angiitis obliterans in the female, migrating phlebitis must be present and must demonstrate the typical microscopic picture at biopsy. All diagnoses lacking the element of migrating phlebitis must be questioned.

[41]

D. Family Incidence.

1. Affects members of the same family but is apparently not inherited. Cases have been reported in enzygotic twins.

   a. The occurrence of thrombo-angiitis obliterans in brothers is quite frequent.

E. Age.

1. Essentially a disease of young men occurring most frequently between the ages of fifteen and forty-five, although cases in older individuals have been observed.

   a. To establish the diagnosis in older patients, there must be evidence of superficial phlebitis, either at the time of examination or in the history obtained from the patient.

   b. Thrombo-angiitis has never been observed in infants or children.

F. Diet.

1. The vasoconstricting action of ergot of rye bread may be an aggravating factor but is not the cause of the disease.

G. Pathology.

1. The inflammatory nature of the disease shows itself by an acute process in the arteries and veins of the extremities, although visceral vessels may also rarely be involved.

2. Artery.

   a. An acute inflammatory reaction in all parts of the arteries as well as the periarterial tissues, with secondary thrombosis of the arterial lumen in which thrombi and giant cells may be found. These cells may also be found in the walls of the arteries or outside the artery.

   b. In the later stages of the disease there is an attempt at healing with thickening and scarring of the arterial wall and canalization and organization of the occluding thrombus.

3. Vein.

   a. The veins show the same acute process described in the arteries.

   b. In the superficial veins of the extremities there is a peculiar migrating type of superficial phlebitis characterized by isolated lengths of superficial veins which become reddened, tender, swollen and palpable. The affected area, which may be one or two inches in length, fades spontaneously after

a few weeks and reappears at some other point along the course of the same or other veins.

c. Any or all extremities may be involved. This type of phlebitis is not accompanied by rise in temperature, by leucocytosis or any generalized symptoms of ordinary phlebitis.

d. Sections of the inflamed superficial vein may be removed under local anesthesia and examined for the characteristic picture, particularly for the giant-cell formation which is pathognomonic of thrombo-angiitis obliterans.

H. Treatment of Migrating Phlebitis.

1. Rest in bed is not essential.

2. Application of a wet dressing of boric acid solution may be used if the phlebitic area becomes painful or tender.

3. A biopsy of the inflamed vein may be made under local anesthesia for diagnostic purposes.

I. Treatment of Thrombo-angiitis Obliterans.

1. Ambulatory treatment.

a. Smoking must be completely eliminated as the vasoconstricting effect is very powerful.

b. Preservation of natural warmth of the extremities by wearing woolen socks and woolen underwear.

(1) This is a much safer method of warming the extremities than the use of external heat such as is obtained from baking lamps or other heating apparatuses.

(2) In severe weather or in climates where the temperature goes very low, wool or felt-lined shoes are also advisable.

c. Hot baths with the water level up to the hips, for ten-minute periods just before retiring are very effective in the production of vasodilatation of the lower extremities. The temperature of the water should not be over 105° F.

(1) The baths are most effective when taken immediately following the postural exercises.

(2) The addition of Epsom salts or other agents to the water is unnecessary as the only benefit from the bath comes from the increased temperature.

d. Short wave treatment.

(1) This is a safe method of improving the collateral circulation in the extremities. Treatments should be given

for twenty-minute periods, three times a week or oftener, depending upon the circumstances.

(a) The patient is allowed to control the intensity of heat in the feet by self-adjustment of the controlling dials. In this way unnecessary discomfort and burns can be avoided.

(b) Remarkable improvement in nail growth may be observed following short wave treatment alone indicating some effects on the circulation in the extremities.

(c) This treatment should be used in conjunction with all other methods.

e. Intravenous injections of 3% or 5% sodium chloride solution, 300 cc., three times a week.

(1) Young vigorous patients may take the 5% solution with no bad after-effects. Some of these may complain of excessive dizziness, in which case the 3% solution should be used. In any case where the 5% concentration is not well tolerated, the 3% or 2% solutions are advisable.

(2) Contraindications to saline therapy are:
  (a) Hypertension.
  (b) Cardiac disease.
  (c) Kidney disease.

(3) Although hypertonic saline solution is available commercially, it may also be prepared by the physician according to the following method:

  (a) Freshly double distilled water must be used.

  (b) To 350 cc. of freshly distilled water, 15, 9, or 6 grams of chemically pure sodium chloride are added depending upon the strength of solution desired.

  (c) The solution is filtered through filter paper.

  (d) The solution is sterilized by boiling for ten minutes over an open flame. It is allowed to cool for twenty-four hours then resterilized for ten minutes by boiling.

  (e) After cooling the solution is injected into the

arm vein by the gravity method using a 19 gauge needle.

(f) If no arm veins are available for the injection, the external jugular may be used.

(g) If the 5% solution causes irritation of the vein at the site of injection the less irritating 3% solution should be used.

(h) Intravenous saline treatment should be given in conjunction with other methods and in the average case should be given for a period of about six months and then once a week for an additional three months.

f. For severe pain of intermittent claudication or severe rest pain intramuscular injections of cobra venom or of de-insulinized pancreatic extract.

(1) Cobra venom is given intramuscularly in doses of 1 cc. once or twice a day as indicated. There are no bad effects following its use.

(2) There are various extracts of pancreas, heart muscle, skeletal muscle, etc., which seem to relieve the pain of intermittent claudication. It cannot be proven that these substances exert any effect upon the peripheral circulation. The tissue extracts may be given in doses of 1 cc. intramuscularly three times a week and may be continued until symptoms improve.

(3) Whiskey in doses of 1 ounce three times a day is a good vasodilator and may relieve pain.

J. Treatment of Impending Gangrene.

1. Absolute rest in bed.

a. This is necessary because thrombo-angiitis obliterans is a generalized infection and when there are open lesions is best treated by complete physiologic rest.

2. Wrapping the entire extremity from the toes to the groin in cotton.

a. External heat in the form of thermostatic cradles, baking lamps and other apparatuses should be scrupulously avoided because of the danger of burns.

3. Prohibition of smoking.

a. This must be complete and uncompromising as the vasoconstrictor action of tobacco cannot be overcome by any known therapeutic agency.

4. Postural exercises.
   a. These should be carried out three or four times a day if practical.
      (1) The legs are elevated at an angle of 45° for approximately two minutes.
      (2) With the patient sitting up the legs hang down for about three minutes.
      (3) With the patient resting the legs are horizontal for two minutes.
      (4) This cycle is repeated four or five times in succession.

5. Hot sitz baths.
   a. The temperature of the bath should not exceed 105° F. and is most effective when taken immediately after the evening exercises.

6. Intravenous injections of hypertonic saline.

7. Intramuscular injections of cobra venom 1 cc. daily.

8. Mechanical apparatuses such as intermittent venous occlusion, suction and pressure machines, oscillating beds, thermostatic cradle, baking apparatuses of all kinds should be avoided in all stages of thrombo-angiitis obliterans because of the vascular damage they may cause.

9. Intravenous injections of typhoid vaccine should be avoided because of the tendency to produce thrombosis of the main vessels during the chill stage of the reaction.

10. Vasodilating drugs are of no benefit in thrombo-angiitis obliterans nor is acetylcholine or its derivatives.
   a. Whiskey three times a day is given for its vasodilating effect.

11. Operative section of sensory nerves for relief of pain in thrombo-angiitis obliterans is an unnecessary and dangerous procedure.
   a. Many chronic ulcers have been caused by the performance of this operation in the poorly nourished tissues of the leg.
   b. Pain in thrombo-angiitis is temporary in character and does not require any operation for its relief.

12. Sympathectomy whether periarterial or of the lumbar ganglia is of temporary if any benefit in thrombo-angiitis obliterans.

a. All cases of thrombo-angiitis obliterans upon whom sympathectomies have been performed have so far shown temporary increase in warmth of the extremities but no permanent improvement in walking or lessening of the chances of gangrene.

K. Indications for Amputation.

1. Destruction of the weight-bearing portion of the foot is the only indication for a major amputation in thrombo-angiitis obliterans. All cases will spontaneously demarcate and heal if proper details of treatment are followed.

L. Local Treatment of Gangrene.

1. Cleanliness is absolutely essential. This is secured by daily bathing of the gangrenous parts in either green soap and water or a ½% solution of chloramine. Following the bath a liberal application of an anesthetic ointment should be applied to the ulcerated area. Of these ointments the following have proven useful:

   a. Nupercainal.

   b. Ethylamino-benzoate ointment 10%.

   c. Panthesin ointment.

   d. Anethaine ointment.

2. Complete bed-rest with the feet on the bed at all times is essential throughout the treatment of gangrene in thrombo-angiitis obliterans.

3. After the acute stage of spreading gangrene and ulceration, if the treatment is carried out properly, a change will take place in the patient's condition. Pain will cease, healthy granulations will appear in the ulcerated area and epithelization will soon start. This may be stimulated by the application of various cod liver oil ointments.

4. If smoking is attempted during the stage of gangrene pain will increase, gangrene will spread and healing will not occur.

M. Complications of Thrombo-angiitis Obliterans.

1. Coronary artery disease in about 10% of the cases.

   a. It has not been determined whether the lesion of the coronary artery is the same as in the extremities.

   b. Many cases of thrombo-angiitis obliterans terminate fatally by thrombosis of the coronary artery.

2. Mesenteric thrombosis.

a. This may result in acute ileus which may prove fatal.

3. Cerebral vascular complications characterized by hemiplegia, aphasia and disturbance of the memory.

4. Secondary infection of gangrenous or ulcerated areas may occur characterized by sudden increase of temperature, lymphangitis of the extremity, chills and malaise. Copious wet dressings to the leg and careful cleansing of the parts locally will soon cause the secondary infection to disappear.

5. Abscesses along the course of the veins of the extremities may occur during the secondary infection. Such abscesses should be incised and drained and penicillin given.

BIBLIOGRAPHY

Allen, E. V.: 'Thrombo-angiitis Obliterans,' *Bull., N. Y. Academy of Med.,* 1942-18-165.

Allen, E. V., and Brown, G. C.: 'Intermittent Pressure and Suction in the Treatment of Chronic Occlusive Arterial Disease,' *J. A. M. A.,* 1935-105-2029.

Barker, N. W.: 'Vasoconstriction Effects of Tobacco Smoking,' *Proc. Staff Meet., Mayo Clin.,* 1932-8-284.

Bernheim, A. R., and London, I. M.: 'Arteriosclerosis and Thrombo-angiitis Obliterans,' *J. A. M. A.,* 1937-108-2102.

Brodie, T. G.: 'The Determination of the Rate of Blood Flow Through an Organ,' *Seventh Internat. Physiol. Cong.,* August, 1907.

Brown, G. E. Allen, E. V., and Mahorner, H. R.: *Thrombo-angiitis Obliterans,* W. B. Saunders Co., 1928.

Bruce, J., Miller, J. R., and Hooker, D. R.: 'The Effect of Smoking upon the Blood Pressure and upon the Volume of the Hand,' *Am. J. Physiol.,* 1909-24-105.

Buerger, L.: *The Circulatory Disturbances of the Extremities,* W. B. Saunders Co., 1924.

Dorsey, J. L.: 'Control of the Tobacco Habit,' *Ann. Int. Med.,* 1936-10-628.

Elliot, A. A., and Nuzum, F. R.: 'The Pharmacologic Properties of an Insulin-Free Extract of Pancreas and the Circulatory Hormone of Frey,' *J. Pharm. & Exp. Ther.,* 1931-43-463.

BIBLIOGRAPHY

Elliot, A. A., and Nuzum, F. R.: 'Pancreatic Extract in the Treatment of Angina Pectoris and Intermittent Claudication,' *Arch. Int. Med.*, 1932-49-1007.

Erb, W.: Über Dysphasia Angiosklerotica intermittierendes Hinken, *München. Med. Wchnschr.*, 1904-51-905.

Frey, E. K., and Kraut, H.: 'Substance Stimulating Heart Activity Excreted by the Kidney,' *Ztschr. f. Biol.*, 1926-84-321.

Ginsburg, N.: 'A Consideration of the Treatment of Peripheral Gangrene Due to Thrombo-angiitis Obliterans,' *Am. J. M. Sc.*, 1917-154-328.

Goodman, C., and Gottesman, J.: 'Pain and Its Treatment in Thrombo-angiitis Obliterans,' *N. Y. Med. J.*, 1923-117-774.

Hausner, E., and Allen, E. V.: 'Generalized Arterial Involvement in Thrombo-angiitis Obliterans including the Report of a Case of Thrombo-angiitis Obliterans of the Pulmonary Artery,' *Proc. Staff Meet., Mayo Clin.*, 1940-15-7.

Horton, B. T.: 'The Outlook in Thrombo-angiitis Obliterans,' *J. A. M. A.*, 1938-11-2184.

Huchard, H.: *Traité clinique des maladies du cœur et de l'aorte*, ed. 3. Paris, Gaston Doin, 1899.

Jablons, B.: 'Thrombo-angiitis Obliterans,' *M. J. & Rec.*, 1924-120-270.

Koga, G.: 'Zur Therapie der Spontangangrän an den Extremitäten,' *Deutsch, Ztschr. f. Chir.*, 1913-121-371.

Kovacs, R., and Kovacs, J.: 'Newer Aspects of Iontophoresis for Arthritis and Circulatory Disturbances,' *Arch. Phys. Therapy, X-ray, Radium*, 1934-15-593.

Lampson, R. S.: 'A Quantitative Study of the Vasoconstriction Induced by Smoking,' *J. A. M. A.*, 1935-104-1963.

Landis, E. M., and Gibbon, J. H., Jr.: 'Effects of Alternate Suction and Pressure on Circulation in the Lower Extremities, *Proc. Soc. Exp. Biol. & Med.*, 1933-30-593.

LeFevre, F. A.: 'Thrombo-angiitis Obliterans,' *Ohio State Med. J.*, 1940-36-272.

Leriche, R.: 'De l'élongation et de la section des nerfs perivasculaires dans certains syndrômes douloureux d'origine artérielle et dans quelques troubles trophique,' *Lyon Chir.*, 1913-10-378.

Maddock, W. G., and Coller, F. A.: 'Peripheral Vasoconstriction by

Tobacco Demonstrated by Skin Temperature Changes,' *Proc. So. Exper. Biol. & Med.*, 1932-29-487.

Maddock, W. G., and Coller, F. A.: 'Peripheral Vasoconstriction of Tobacco and Its Relation to Thrombo-angiitis Obliterans,' *Ann. Surg.*, 1933-98-70.

Major, R. T., and Cline, J. K.: 'Preparation and Properties of Alpha- and Beta-methylcholine and Gamma-homocholine,' *J. Am. Chem. Soc.*, 1932-54-242.

Mayesima, J.: 'Klinische u. experimentelle Untersuchungen über die Viscosität des Blutes,' *Mitt. a. d. Grenzgeb. d. Med. u. Chir.*, 1911-24-413.

Meyer, W.: 'The Conservative Treatment of Gangrene of the Extremities Due to Thrombo-angiitis Obliterans,' *Ann. Surg.*, 1916-63-280.

Michels, E.: 'Uber angiosklerotische Gangrän bei jugendlichen Individuen,' *Klin. Jahrb.*, 1909-21-557.

Mohs, F. E., Sevringhaus, E. L., and Schmidt, E. R.: 'Conservative Amputation of Gangrenous Parts by Chemosurgery,' *Ann. Surg.*, 1941-Vol. 114-274.

Nemec, K.: 'Experiments on Danger of Air Embolism in Intravenous Injection,' *Klin. Jahrb.*, 1909-21-557.

Reid, M. R., and Herrmann, L. G.: 'Treatment of Obliterative Vascular Diseases by Means of an Intermittent Negative Pressure Environment,' *J. Med.*, 1933-14-200.

Samuels, S. S.: 'Treatment of Gangrene Due to Thrombo-angiitis Obliterans,' *J. A. M. A.*, 1931-96-751.

'Gangrene Due to Thrombo-angiitis Obliterans, Further Experiences with Treatment,' *J. A. M. A.*, 1934-102-436.

'The Conservative Treatment of Thrombo-angiitis Obliterans,' *Lancet*, 1936-2-1511.

'Peripheral Arterial Diseases—The Fundamentals in Their Diagnosis and Treatment,' *J. M. Soc. New Jersey*, 1938-35-224.

Samuels, S. S., Ferber, J., and Weichsel, H.: 'Rationale of Saline Therapy, *Lucien Howe Prize Essay, Med. Soc. State of N. Y.*, 1933.

Schwartzman, M. S.: 'Muscle Extract in Treatment of Angina Pectoris and Intermittent Claudication,' *Brit. M. J.*, 1930-1-855.

Silbert, S.: 'The Treatment of Thrombo-angiitis Obliterans by Intra-

venous Injection of Hypertonic Salt Solution,' *J. A. M. A.,* 1926-86-1759.

Simici, D., and Marcu, I.: 'Récherches pléthysmographiques sur l'action vasculaire de la fumée de tabac chez l'homme, *Bull. et Mém. Soc. Méd. de Hôp. de Bucarest,* 1926-8-233.

Steel, W. A.: 'Sodium Citrate Treatment of Thrombo-angiitis Obliterans,' *Med. Rec.,* 1921-76-429.

Thienes, C. H., and Butt, E. M.: 'Chronic Circulatory Effects of Tobacco and Nicotine,' *Am. J. M. Sc.,* 1938-48-258.

Theis, F. V., and Freeland, M. R.: 'Thrombo-angiitis Obliterans: Treatment with Sodium Tetrothionate and Sodium Thiosulfate,' *Arch. Surg.,* 1940-40-190.

'Thrombo-angiitis Obliterans: Clinical Observations and Arterial Blood Oxygen Studies During Treatment of Disease with Sodium Tetrothionate and Sodium Thiosulfate,' *Surgery,* 1942-11-101.

Weiss, S.: 'Arteritis: Diseases Associated with Inflammatory Lesions of Peripheral Arteries,' *New Eng. J. of Med.,* 1941-225-579.

Wolffe, J. B., Findlay, D., and Dessen, E.: 'Treatment of Angina Pectoris with Tissue Vasodilating Extract—preliminary report,' *Ann. Int. Med.,* 1931-5-625.

Wright, I. S., and Moffatt, D.: 'The Effects of Tobacco on the Peripheral Vascular System,' *J. A. M. A.,* 1934-103-318.

VIII

RAYNAUD'S DISEASE

A. Etiology.
  1. Endocrine disturbance.
    a. This has been suspected, but not proven.
  2. Metabolic disorders.
    a. May be the cause.
  3. Infection.
    a. Unlikely.
B. Pathology.
  1. Distribution.
    a. Open question as to whether the disease is a local fault of the peripheral arterioles or, as originally described by Raynaud, a disturbance of the sympathetic nervous system.
C. Symptoms.
  1. Distribution.
    a. Symmetrical involvement of all extremities in episodes of vasomotor disturbance characterized by blanching of the fingers and toes which in turn is followed by deep cyanosis and rubor with return to normal color after a short time.
  2. Direct causes.
    a. Attacks may be initiated by exposure to cold or by emotional upset.
    b. Residence in a warm climate does not cure the disease as attacks may be brought on by emotional factors.
  3. Gangrenous ulcers.
    a. Ulcers of the tips of the fingers may occur in advanced stages of the disease.
      (1) These ulcers are extremely painful and cause great disability because of the patient's loss of the use of the fingers. They seldom become secondarily infected and yield to treatment quite easily.

4. Sex distribution.

    a. More prevalent in women but many cases have been observed in men.

5. Excessive perspiration.

    a. May affect hands and feet.

6. Hemoglobinuria.

    a. This may be present but is not constant.

7. Transient aphasia.

    a. Paralysis or amblyopia may be present.

8. Scleroderma

    a. This may affect the extremities and face. Many also have rheumatoid arthritis of the hands.

    b. The scleroderma may be very mild or it may be so severe as to interfere with writing and may produce a mask-like expression of the face. When occurring on the chest it may interfere with breathing.

    c. The arthritic condition of the hands is usually very painful and disabling and may be associated with swelling of the joints of the fingers.

D. Treatment.

  1. Warmth.

    a. Avoidance of exposure to cold is very important.

      (1) The use of warm gloves and woolen stockings is essential during cold weather. Woolen underwear is also advisable.

      (2) The use of external heat such as thermostatic cradles and baking lamps should be avoided as the danger of burns is great and excessive heat may cause attacks of spasm in the same way as excessive cold.

    b. A daily hot bath is very valuable.

      (1) The bath is most effective if taken just before retiring. The temperature should not be over 105° F.

    c. Short wave diathermy.

      (1) This may be given to all extremities for twenty-minute periods three times a week.

  2. Iontophoresis with mecholyl (acetyl-beta-methylcholine chloride).

    a. Mecholyl may be given orally in the form of tablets of mecholyl bromide 0.20 GM (gr. iii) one or two tablets twice a day or it may be given subcutaneously in the form of mecholyl chloride 0.025 GM or by iontophoresis.

   (1) In giving the drug by iontophoresis, $\frac{1}{10}$ to $\frac{1}{2}\%$ solution in saline is used by saturating asbestos paper and applying it under the positive galvanic pole. The treatment is carried out for twenty minutes using 20 to 30 milliamperes.

3. Acetylcholine.
   a. Acetylcholine is decomposed immediately upon its injection into living tissue.

4. Hypertonic saline injections.
   a. 300 cc. of 2, 3 or 5% saline, depending upon the age and general condition of the patient, can be given three times a week for six months to a year. This should be used in conjunction with other methods of therapy.

5. Vasodilators.
   a. Nitroglycerine and amyl nitrite have been used but with poor results.
      (1) Phenacetin or aspirin may help in the relief of pain.
      (2) Morphine and opium derivatives should be avoided if possible as they have a mild vasoconstricting action.
   b. Alcoholic beverages have a good vasodilating effect.

6. Sympathectomy may be tried but the results are not as beneficial as were expected.
   a. The operation must be complete if it is to be beneficial.
   b. Preliminary studies should be made to determine whether or not the distal vessels can be dilated.
   c. Better results have been obtained in the lower extremities than in the upper.
   d. In the presence of scleroderma the operation should not be done.

7. Gangrenous lesions and ulcerations of the fingertips may be treated by cleanliness, daily baths with the application of a soothing ointment.
   a. The parts should be dressed daily and bland ointments should be used. Boric acid ointment should be tried. If this is painful various anesthetic ointments should be the next choice.
   b. Complete bed-rest is essential.

8. Intermittent venous compression and other mechanical methods of treatment are useless.

E. Prognosis.

1. Mild cases may not change over a period of years.

2. Cases with scleroderma and arthritis usually become worse in spite of all treatment and may end fatally with pneumonia or other complications.

BIBLIOGRAPHY

Allen, E. V., and Brown, G. E.: 'Raynaud's Disease: a clinical study of one hundred and forty-seven cases,' *J. A. M. A.,* 1932-99-1472.

Allen, E. V.: 'Peripheral Arteries in Raynaud's Disease: arteriographic study of living subjects,' *Proc. Staff Meet., Mayo Clin.,* 1937-12-187.

Cassirer, R.: *Die vasomotorisch-trophischen Neurosen,* Berlin, S. Karger, 1912.

Duryee, A. W., and Wright, I. S.: 'Studies of Human Capillaries,' *Am. J. M. Sc.,* 1933-185-664.

Guedjian, E. S., and Walker, L. W., 'Traumatic Vasospastic Disease of the Hand (White Fingers),' *J. A. M. A.,* 1945-10-668.

Homans, J.: *Circulatory Diseases of the Extremities,* The Macmillan Co., 1939.

Johnson, C. A.: 'Study of Clinical Manifestations and Results of Treatment of Twenty-two Patients with Raynaud's Symptoms,' *Surg. Gynec. & Obst.,* Chicago, 1941-72-889.

Kraetzer, A. F.: 'Raynaud's Disease: hypothesis as to its cause,' *N. Y. State J. Med.,* 1935-35-1130.

Lewis, T.: 'Experiments Relating to the Peripheral Mechanism Involved in Spasmodic Arrest of the Circulation in the Fingers, a Variety of Raynaud's Disease,' *Heart,* 1929-15-7.

'Further Observations upon a Variety of Raynaud's Disease: with special reference to arteriolar defects and to scleroderma,' *Heart,* 1931-16-33.

The Blood Vessels of the Human Skin and Their Responses, London, 1927, Shaw & Sons.

Vascular Disorders of the Limbs, The Macmillan Co., 1936.

Mueller, O.: 'Die Kapillaren der menschlichen Körperoberfläche in Gesunden u. Kranken,' *Enke,* Stuttgart, 1922.

O'Leary, P. A., and Waisman, M.: 'Acrosclerosis,' *Proc. Staff Meet., Mayo Clin.,* 1940-15-702.

Raynaud, M.: 'De l'asphyxie locale et de la gangrène symétrique des extrémitiés,' *Arch. gén. de Méd.,* 1874-1-5.

Selected Monographs. On Local Asphyxia and Symmetrical Gangrene of the Extremities, London, *The New Sydenham Society,* 1888-121-1.

Redisch, W.: 'Zur Kapillarmikroskopie und Kapillarphotographie,' *Zeitschr. f. Kreislaufforschung,* 1930-22-39.

Wertheimer, P., and Bérard, M.: 'A propos de la maladie de Raynaud. Considérations thérapeutiques et pathologiques d'après 13 observations,' *J. de Chir.,* 1938-52-737.

White, J. C.: *The Autonomic Nervous System,* The Macmillan Co., 1935.

IX

ERYTHROMELALGIA

A. Clinical Picture.
1. Described by Weir Mitchell in 1870, apparently a disturbance of the vasodilating mechanism causing burning pain in the extremities, increase in local heat of the affected parts, aggravation of the attack by exertion and relief of symptoms by rest and application of cold or cold environment and elevation of the affected extremity. Oscillometric readings increase during an attack.

B. Etiology.
1. Unknown.
2. Extremely rare.
3. No special age group.
4. May affect either sex.
5. Usually affects the lower extremities but cases have been described in the upper extremities.
   a. May affect an isolated extremity.

C. Symptoms.
1. Gradual onset.
2. Attacks initiated by heat, exercises, dependency of the extremities.

D. Physical Signs.
1. Increased heat of the extremity.
2. Increased arterial pulsation.
   a. Oscillometric index increased during an attack.
3. Excessive redness of the skin of the involved extremity during an attack.

E. Diagnosis.
1. Must be differentiated from arteriosclerosis and thrombo-angiitis obliterans.

F. Treatment.
1. There is no successful treatment so far as known.

2. Elevation of the extremity and application of cold usually give temporary relief.

3. Spontaneous disappearance of all symptoms has been observed.

BIBLIOGRAPHY

Brown, G. E.: 'Erythromelalgia and Other Disturbances of the Extremities Accompanied by Vasodilatation and Burning,' *Am. J. M. Sc.,* 1932-183-468.

Cassirer, R.: *Die vasomotorisch-trophischen Neurosen,* Berlin, S. Karger, 1912.

Lewis, T.: 'Clinical Observations and Experiments Relating to Burning Pain in Extremities and to So-called "Erythromelalgia" in Particular,' *Cl. Science,* 1933-1-175.

Mitchell, S. W.: 'Clinical Lecture on Certain Painful Affections of the Feet,' *Philadelphia Med. Times,* 1872-3-81.

'On a Rare Vasomotor Neurosis of the Extremities, and on the Maladies with Which It May Be Conformed,' *Am. J. M. Sc.,* 1878-76-17.

Mufson, I.: 'Clinical Observations in Erythromelalgia and a Method for Its Symptomatic Relief,' *Am. Heart J.,* 1937-13-483.

Saracoglu, K. S.: 'Rare Case of Erythromelalgia,' *Schw. med. Wchnsch.,* 1939-69-607.

Smith, L. A., and Allen, E. V.: 'Erthermalgia (erythromelalgia) of Extremities; syndrome characterized by redness, heat, and pain,' *Am. Heart J.,* 1938-16-175.

X

ACROCYANOSIS

A. Clinical Picture.
1. Persistent purplish discoloration of the hands or feet or of both upper and lower extremities simultaneously.
2. No cycle of color changes, merely a persistence of cyanosis.

B. Etiology.
1. No definite etiologic factor is known.
2. The disease is more prevalent in young women but men may also be affected.
   a. There may be a sudden onset at puberty.
   b. In older individuals the onset may be gradual.
3. Endocrine disturbances may be present.
4. The cyanosis which usually extends to the wrists or ankles may be intensified by cold or psychic influences.
5. Excessive perspiration of the hands and feet is the rule.
   a. Hands may be indurated or puffy.
   b. Paresthesias may be present.

C. Diagnosis.
1. Must be distinguished from Raynaud's disease, arteriosclerosis obliterans and thrombo-angiitis obliterans.

D. Treatment.
1. Retention of natural warmth of the extremities by warm covering.
2. Hot baths.
3. Short wave diathermy.
4. Vasodilator drugs or thyroid substance may be tried.
5. Sympathetic ganglionectomy is too formidable an operation for this minor disturbance.

BIBLIOGRAPHY

Barker, N. W., and Baker, G. S.: 'Acrocyanosis: Effect of Cervico-thoracic Sympathectomy: Report of a Case,' *Proc. Staff Meet., Mayo Clin.,* 1940-15-601.

Cassirer, R.: *Die vasomotorisch-trophischen Neurosen,* Berlin, S. Karger, 1912.

Groom, R. J.: 'Acrodynia,' *Rocky Mountain M. J.,* 1941-38-616.

Layani, F.: *Les Acrocynoses,* Paris, Masson, 1929.

XI

EMBOLISM

A. Etiology.
1. The usual cause is detachment of thrombi from the walls or valves of the left side of the heart. Mural thrombi are frequently found in auricular fibrillation.
2. Another source of emboli is a mural thrombus of the left ventricle following an attack of coronary artery closure.
3. A less frequent source of embolus is from a calcified, ulcerated plaque on the aorta or other large vessel. Paradoxical emboli usually arise from thrombosed veins of an extremity and are carried through a patent foramen ovale to the left side of the heart where they cause embolic phenomena in the limbs.

B. Predisposing Causes.
1. Auricular fibrillation, particularly when there is a transition to normal heart rhythm.
2. Occlusion of the coronary artery with thrombosis of the walls of the heart (aneurysm of the heart).
3. Acute or subacute bacterial endocarditis, usually the former.

C. Sites of Lodgment of Emboli.
1. At the bifurcation of the aorta into the iliac artery (saddle embolus).
2. At the origin of the profunda femoral.
3. At the bifurcation of the popliteal into the anterior and posterior tibials.
4. In the upper extremities most usual site for lodgment of an embolus is in the axillary artery.

D. Symptoms.
1. Usually sudden onset with severe pain in the affected extremity plus ischemia; subjective coldness of the extremity also noted.
   a. Other symptoms that may be noted when there is sudden closure of the larger arteries are nausea and vomiting and symptoms of shock. This syndrome, however, is quite rare.

2. After a few hours, cyanosis of the affected part sets in which may progress within forty-eight hours or longer to gangrene of the extremity.

3. Soon after the embolic phenomena has occurred the extremity becomes extremely pale and cold. The coldness is usually sharply demarcated at the point where the arterial circulation changes. There is loss of pulsation in the arteries distal to the point of lodgment of the embolus. This may be detected either by palpation or more accurately with the oscillometer.

    a. Histamine test and wheal test are not reliable to determine the level of obstruction.

    b. Anesthesia, paresis and loss of reflexes may also be present in the involved extremity.

    c. Secondary vasospasm in the involved limb may be present to some degree but plays only a minor role in the clinical picture.

E. Treatment.

1. Preservation of the natural warmth of the extremity by wrapping it completely in cotton.

    a. The cotton should be kept on continuously and should not be disturbed except for daily inspection of the parts.

    b. External heat in the form of baking lamps or thermostatic cradles should be avoided as serious burns may be produced.

    c. Secondary vasospasm is overcome to a great degree by wrapping the extremities in cotton.

2. Complete bed-rest.

    a. This is very essential and should be continued until complete resolution of the process has occurred.

    b. The limbs should be held in the horizontal position at all times.

3. Papaverine or intramuscular injections of cobra venom for relief of pain.

    a. Papaverine may be given intravenously, subcutaneously or orally three to four times per day.

    b. Cobra venom is given in doses of 1 cc. intramuscularly once or twice a day depending upon the severity of the symptoms.

4. Vasodilator drugs such as the nitrites may be given but are usually of no value.

a. Amyl nitrite may be used as a vasodilator.

b. Acetylcholine and its derivatives are of no avail in this condition.

5. Suction—pressure and intermittent venous compression therapy have proven not only valueless but may spread the process. Therefore they are not to be used.

6. Heparin may be given intravenously. 10 milligrams or 1,000 units, added to each 100 cc. of saline solution, is allowed to drip into the vein at the rate of about 25 drops per minute, maintaining the clotting time at about 15 minutes. Heparin treatment should be continued for about 10 days, if possible.

   a. Dicumarol therapy is too uncertain to be used routinely because of the difficulty in controlling its effects.

7. Embolectomy to be successful must be performed within six hours of the onset of the accident.

   a. The operation is performed under local anesthesia and successful results have been obtained in about 50% of the cases operated upon.

   b. The operation does not eliminate the possibility of recurrence of embolism in some other part of the body.

   c. Heparin therapy should be administered before and after operation and should be continued for about 10 days.

8. If a line of demarcation forms in the foot and leaves the weight-bearing part of the extremity intact, conservative treatment may be continued. If the resulting gangrene destroys the weight-bearing portion of extremity amputation must be done.

   a. In the upper extremities greater conservatism should be practiced than in the lower since the collateral circulation in the upper extremities is normally much greater than in the lower and the indiscriminate amputation of a hand or arm is of much greater consequence.

   b. Quite often after waiting a sufficiently long time with conservative treatment the gangrenous process will demarcate itself to individual digits of either extremity. When such demarcation has occurred, mummification will follow and the gangrenous parts should be carefully removed, allowing the stump to heal spontaneously. In this way the patient may come through with the loss of only part of one or more digits and thus be spared a major amputation.

BIBLIOGRAPHY

Denk, W.: 'Zur Behandlung der arteriellen Embolie,' *München. med. Wchnschr.*, 1934-81-437.

'Weitere Erfahrungen mit der unblutigen Behandlung der Embolie,' *Zentralbl. f. Chir.*, 1936-63-2.

Funck-Brentano, P.: 'Differential Diagnosis of Arterial Embolism of Members,' *Presse Méd.*, 1939-47-1569.

Haimovici, H.: *Les Embolies artérielles des membres*, Paris, Masson, 1937.

Les Occlusions artérielles aigües des membres, Paris, Masson, 1939.

Jorpes, J. E.: *Heparin: Its Chemistry, Physiology and Application in Medicine*, Oxford University Press, N. Y. and London, 1939.

Key, E.: 'Über Embolektomie als Behandlungsmethode bei embolischen Zirkulationsstörungen der Extremitäten,' *Acta Chir. Scandinavica*, 1922-54-339.

'Sur l'embolectomie comme méthode de traitement des troubles de la circulation par embolie des extrémités,' *Lyon Chir.*, 1923-20-1.

'L'embolectomie dans les Troubles embolique des Extrémités,' *Lyon Chir.*, 1928-25-269.

'Die Embolie Operationen auf Grund des bisherigen Erfahrungen,' *Ergebn. d. Chir. u. Orthop.*, 1929-22-1.

'Embolectomy of the Vessels of the Extremities,' *Brit. J. Surg.*, 1936-24-350.

Link, C. P., et al.: 'Studies on the Hemorrhagic Sweet Clover Disease,' *J. Biol. Chem.*, 1940-136-47; ibid., 1941-138-1; 1941-138-21; 1941-138-513.

Loewe, L., Rosenblatt, P., and Hirsch, E.: 'Use of Heparin in Treatment of Venous Thromboembolic Disease,' *J. A. M. A.*, 1946-130-386.

McKechnie, R. E., and Allen, E. V.: 'Sudden Occlusion of the Arteries of the Extremities: a study of 100 cases of embolism and thrombosis,' *Proc. Staff Meet., Mayo Clin.*, 1935-10-673.

Nystrom, G.: 'Zur Prognose und Methodik der Embolektomie,' *Zentralbl. f. Chir.*, 1926-53-1.

Pratt, G. H.: 'Surgical Management of Acute Arterial Occlusion,' *J. A. M. A.*, 1946-130-827.

XII

CERVICAL RIB AND SCALENUS ANTICUS SYNDROME

A. Definition.
  1. Cervical rib is a congenital anomaly whereby an extra rib which may be only rudimentary is found above the normal first thoracic rib opposite the seventh cervical vertebra.
     a. This condition may be familial.
     b. Either sex may be affected but it is supposed to be more prominent in women.
B. Etiology.
  1. The etiology of the scalenus anticus syndrome is a fibrous thickening of the posterior portion of the scalenus anticus muscle. This is also a developmental anomaly.
C. Symptoms.
  1. Both conditions are the same and are caused by pressure of either the rib and its fibrous extension or a fibrosis of the scalenus anticus muscle upon either the brachial plexus or the subclavian artery.
  2. Symptoms do not as a rule appear until after adolescence.
  3. Pressure on the brachial plexus causes symptoms in the ulnar distribution.
  4. Pain or a dull ache may be felt in either the hands, arms, shoulder or neck.
  5. Paresthesias also may be present.
  6. Muscular weakness of the affected extremity together with wasting of the small muscles of the hand and sometimes of the flexors of the arm are occasionally seen.
  7. Vascular symptoms.
     a. These are usually spastic in nature resembling those of Raynaud's disease. Thrombosis of the subclavian artery is also possible.
     b. The vascular effects are intensified by drawing the arm forcibly down to the side, pulling it backward or raising it far above the head.

        (1) Oscillometry will show diminished pulsation with this maneuver.

    c. Vascular signs.

        (1) Coldness of the hands or fingers.

        (2) Cyanosis and decrease in the radial and ulnar or both pulsations as revealed by the oscillometer.

    d. Gangrene of the fingers may occur.

        (1) Thrombosis of the subclavian artery may occur.

8. Neurologic symptoms.

    a. Motor symptoms.

        (1) Weakness.

        (2) Atrophy.

        (3) Reaction of degeneration.

        (4) Paralysis has also been observed.

    b. Sensory symptoms.

        (1) Pain.

        (2) Paresthesia.

    c. Vasomotor changes.

        (1) Cyanosis.

        (2) Edema.

        (3) Coldness.

        (4) These symptoms may be partly due to pressure on the vascular system.

        (5) Cervical sympathetic paralysis.

9. Roentgen examination may show the accessory rib which may be bilateral.

    a. A negative roentgen examination does not exclude scalenus anticus syndrome nor the presence of a fibrous rib not visible by x-ray.

D. Treatment.

1. Mild cases, elevation of the shoulder by bandages or by a temporary cast is sufficient.

2. Where these do not give success, removal of the cervical rib or cutting the fibrous band of the scalenus anticus muscle is necessary.

    a. The operation for dividing the scalenus anticus muscle is performed as follows, under local anesthesia:

        (1) Skin incision one inch above and parallel with clav-

icle to lateral edge of sternomastoid—about two inches long.

(2) Avoid cutting the external jugular vein.

(3) Divide the platysma.

(4) Retract the clavicular part of the sternomastoid medially.

(5) Cut or retract the posterior belly of the omohyoid.

(6) Isolate the scalenus anticus with a retractor.

(7) Completely cut the scalenus anticus muscle.

(8) Close wound with small drain using silk for sutures.

BIBLIOGRAPHY

Belgrano, M.: 'Cervical Ribs: Clinical and X-ray Study,' *Giorn. Veneto d. Sci. Med.*, 1940-14-155.

Hill, R. M.: 'Vascular Anomalies of Upper Limbs Associated with Cervical Ribs: Report of a Case and Review of Literature,' *Brit. J. Surg.*, 1939-27-100.

Jones, R., and Lovett, R. W.: *Orthopedic Surgery*, Wm. Wood & Co., 1929.

MacFee, W. F.: 'Cervical Rib Causing Partial Occlusion and Aneurysm of Subclavian Artery,' *Ann. Surg.*, 1940-111-549.

Patterson, R. H.: 'Cervical Ribs and Scalenus Muscle Syndrome, *Ann. Surg.*, 1940-111-531.

Smith, B. C.: 'Thrombosis of Third Portion of Subclavian Artery Associated with Scalenus Anticus Syndrome,' *Ann. Surg.*, 1940-111-546.

Spurling, R. G., and Bradford, F. K.: 'Scalenus Neurocirculatory Compression,' *Ann. Surg.*, 1938-107-708.

Theis, F. V.: 'Scalenus Anticus Syndrome and Cervical Ribs,' *Surgery*, 1939-6-112.

XIII

AXILLARY VEIN THROMBOSIS

A. Etiology.
1. It is usually traumatic, caused by lifting heavy objects or forceful motion of the shoulder joints.
    a. Usually more affected in the left.
    b. More common in males although cases have been seen in females.

B. Symptoms.
1. Enlargement of the affected extremity with increase in temperature of the hand and fingers.
2. Axillary vein felt as a hard tender cord which easily rolls under the examining finger.
3. More distally distributed veins of the arm dilated and **do not** collapse upon elevation of the arm above the head.
    a. Venograms are helpful in diagnosis.

C. Treatment.
1. Complete rest with wet dressings in acute phase.
    a. Heparin intravenous drip may be beneficial.
2. Short wave diathermy later.
3. Compression with a semi-elastic bandage may be used in the late stages if edema is present.

BIBLIOGRAPHY

Foster, R., Brouwer, S. W., and Kurtz, C. M.: 'Thrombosis of the Inferior Vena Cava following Physical Exertion,' *J. A. M. A.,* 1941-117-2167.

Kaplan, T.: 'Thrombosis of the Axillary Vein,' *J. A. M. A.,* 1938-110-2059.

Von Schröter: *Nothnagel's Handbuch der Pathologie u. Therapie,* 1884.

XIV

FROST-BITE (THERMAL GANGRENE)

A. Etiology.
1. Caused by exposure to cold.

B. Symptoms.
1. In mild cases persistent ischemia of the fingers, hands, nose and feet accompanied by numbness and tingling or anesthesia of the parts.
2. Advanced cases may develop gangrene.

C. Treatment.
1. Prophylaxis is important.
2. Complete rest, maintaining the warmth of the extremities by wrapping in cotton or lamb's wool.
   a. The wearing of warm, dry clothing in cold, windy weather is essential.
   b. If exposure to cold is unavoidable it should be for brief periods only.
   c. The protective covering should be kept on continuously until the entire process has resolved.
3. Warm sitz baths.
   a. These may be given daily for ten-minute periods with the temperature of the water not over 100° F.
4. In the presence of gangrene, daily foot baths in green soap and water followed by wet dressing of boric acid solution to cause maceration and separation of the gangrenous parts.
   a. The remaining stump covered with granulation tissue may then be treated with boric acid ointment or cod-liver oil ointment to stimulate healing.
   b. In some extensive cases skin grafts may be necessary.
   c. Major amputation of limbs should not be done until conservative therapy has been given a thorough trial.

BIBLIOGRAPHY

Brahdy, L.: 'Frostbites among Employees of the City of New York,' *J. A. M. A.*, 1935-104-529.

DeTakats, G.: *Chapter on Trauma and Peripheral Vascular Disease in Brahdy and Kahn, Trauma and Disease,* Lea & Febiger, 1937.

Kaplan, T.: 'Frost-Bite,' *Am. J. Surg.*, 1936-32-318.

Lange, K., and Loewe, L.: 'Subcutaneous Heparin in Pitkin Menstruum for Treatment of Experimental Human Frostbite,' *Surg. Gyn. & Obs.*, 1946-82-256.

Leriche, R., and Kunlin, J.: 'Pathologic Physiology of Frost-Bites: Vasomotor and Thrombotic Disease,' *Progrès. Méd.*, Paris, 1940-68-169.

XV

GLOMUS TUMOR

A. Clinical Picture.
1. Glomus is a short-cut communication between the arterial and venous side of the circulation for regulation of superficial body temperature.
    a. When this anastomosis becomes hypertrophied it is known as a glomus tumor.
2. It may occur in any portion of the body but is usually under the fingernail.
3. There is a tiny elevation surrounded by bluish or reddish discoloration.
4. The nodules are extremely tender.
    a. May be induced by trauma.
5. They usually occur in early adult life.
6. The glomus tumor may pulsate.
7. May be local elevation of skin temperature.
8. The slightest pressure or even contact with clothing may cause excruciating pain.

B. Treatment.
1. Complete excision under local anesthesia is the only satisfactory method.
2. Radiotherapy may be tried but is usually unsuccessful.

BIBLIOGRAPHY

Adair, F. E.: 'Glomus Tumor,' *Am. J. Surg.*, 1934-25-1.

Bailey, O. T.: 'The Cutaneous Glomus and Its Tumors—Glomangiomas,' *Am. J. Path.*, 1935-11-915.

Blanchard, A. J.: 'Pathology of Glomus Tumors,' *Can. Med. Ass. J.*, Montreal, 1941-44-357.

Blinder, S.: 'Glomus Tumor,' *Am. Heart J.*, 1939-17-238.

Hoffman, H. O. E., and Ghormley, R. K.: 'Glomus Tumor and Intramuscular Lipoma: Report of Two Cases,' *Proc. Staff Meet., Mayo Clin.*, 1941-16-13.

Pleeves, B.: 'Multiple Glomus Tumors: Four In One Finger,' *Can. Med. Ass. J.,* Montreal, 1941-44-364.

Popoff, N. W.: 'The Digital Vascular System,' *Arch. Path.,* 1934-18-295.

Sucquet, J.: Cited by Popoff.

XVI

ANEURYSM OF PERIPHERAL VESSELS

A. Simple Aneurysm of the Extremities.
  1. Etiology.
      a. Almost always traumatic in origin.
  2. Diagnosis.
      a. Pulsating swelling in the neighborhood of the main vessel.
      b. In some cases interference with the blood flow of the affected artery may cause symptoms in the extremity such as:
          (1) Intermittent claudication.
          (2) Ischemia.
          (3) Coldness.
      c. Simple aneurysm may rupture causing large extravasations of blood or external hemorrhage which may be fatal.
  3. Treatment.
      a. Extirpation of the aneurysm or, if possible, ligation of the artery above the aneurysm may be performed.

B. Arteriovenous Aneurysm.
  1. Etiology.
      a. Abnormal communications between the large arteries and veins of the extremities are usually traumatic in origin although they may be congenital.
  2. Symptoms and signs.
      a. Enlargement of the extremity.
      b. Signs of unusual pressure in the veins of the affected limb, such as:
          (1) Engorgement resembling varicosities.
          (2) Visible or palpable pulsation of the veins.
          (3) Increased temperature in the entire extremity.
          (4) Peculiar reddish color of the superficial veins due to the presence of arterial blood.
          (5) Loud bruit or thrill may be heard over the superficial vessels.
          (6) Bruit may be heard in the opposite extremity.

(7) Other symptoms of arteriovenous aneurysm:
   (a) Low arterial blood pressure.
   (b) Increased pulse rate.
   (c) Enlargement of the heart.
   (d) Cardiac decompensation.
   (e) Gangrene of distal parts may also occur.
   (f) Arteriography a valuable diagnostic procedure.

3. Treatment.
   a. Obliteration of the large varicose veins by injection method.
   b. Exposure of the fistula by incision through the venous or arterial wall.
   c. Separation of the vessels and ligation of all communicating branches.
   d. Excision of both vessels at the site of the fistula.

BIBLIOGRAPHY

Aguiar, J. A., and Lima, M. F. V.: 'Spontaneous Aneurysm of Subclavian Artery Case,' *Brasil-Med.,* 1940-54-2.

Holman, E.: *Arteriovenous Aneurysm,* The Macmillan Co., 1937.

Libman, E.: Cases of Mycotic Aneurysms, *Mt. Sinai Hosp.,* Rep., 1905-06-5-481.

Smith, F. L., and Horton, B. T.: 'Sclerosing Treatment of Congenital Arteriovenous Fistula,' *Proc. Staff Meet., Mayo Clin.,* 1937-12-17.

Theis, F. F.: 'Popliteal Aneurysms as a Cause of Peripheral Circulatory Disease: With Special Study of Oscillomographs as an Aid to Diagnosis,' *Surgery,* 1927-2-327.

Waugh, J. M., and Neel, H. B.: 'Traumatic Arteriovenous Fistula of the Femoral Vessels: Report of a Case,' *Proc. Staff Meet., Mayo Clin.,* 1941-16-134.

XVII

VARICOSE VEINS

A. Definition.

1. Varicose veins are dilated, sometimes fibrosed veins with incompetent valves, with deficiency and inability to carry blood as part of the return circulation.

   a. They are most common in the legs and are usually superficial.

B. Etiology.

1. Hereditary factors.
2. Pregnancy.
3. Prolonged standing.
4. Over-exertion.
5. Endocrine influence.

C. Symptoms.

1. May be absent entirely.
2. Heavy feeling in legs.
3. Paresthesias of skin of lower extremities.
4. Edema of legs and ankles.

D. Diagnosis.

1. Trendelenburg test.

   a. The leg to be examined is elevated for a moment or two and a tourniquet passed firmly around the midthigh after the superficial veins are emptied.

   b. The leg is now depressed and if the superficial veins below the tourniquet fill rapidly the communicating veins of the leg are incompetent.

2. Perthes test.

   a. A modification of the Trendelenburg test to test incompetency of the deep veins of the legs. A tourniquet is applied above the knee and the patient walks about for a few moments. If with the tourniquet in place the veins below do not distend after the patient walks about, the deep venous system of the leg is competent.

E. Treatment.

  1. Palliative measures such as the application of elastic bandages or rubber stockings.

  2. Obliteration of veins by injection of chemicals.

   a. Sclerosing chemicals.

    (1) Sodium morrhuate 5%.

    (2) Quinine hydrochloride and urethane.

    (3) 50% glucose.

    (4) 10% or 20% sodium chloride.

    (5) Sodium tetradecyl sulfate 3%.

  3. Technic of injection.

   a. A fine hypodermic needle is used with a 2 cc. syringe. The most distally dilated veins are injected first.

   b. With the leg in the dependent position the overlying skin is sterilized with alcohol and about 1 cc. of the solution is injected into the varicosity at its lowermost point.

   c. When the vein is entered accurately, as is shown by a back-flow of blood into the syringe, the material is injected slowly and as soon as the needle is removed from the vein a sterile pad is applied and an elastic bandage immediately used.

   d. This is kept in place for twenty-four hours. Successive injections may be given at intervals of two or three days depending upon the severity of the reaction.

   e. It is not necessary to obliterate every varicose vein in the leg, only the most prominent should be treated.

   f. The treatment is ambulatory and should not interfere with the patient's occupation.

  4. Litigation of internal saphenous vein.

   a. In cases of extreme dilatation and incompetence of the internal saphenous vein, resection of the vein at its point of entry into the femoral vein should be done under local anesthesia. Postoperative injection of the varicosities is preferable.

  5. Varicose ulcer.

   a. A common complication of varicose veins together with varicose eczema.

    (1) Etiology.

     (a) In the vast percentage of cases the ulcer is ini-

tiated by a tinea infection which thrives in the poorly nourished tissues of the leg. This is probably also the cause of many cases of varicose eczema. As the ulcer enlarges the tinea infection together with the poor nutrition of the tissues serves to keep the ulcer open and chronic.

(2) Treatment of varicose ulcer.

(a) Improvement of local nutrition by either obliteration of all varicosities in the immediate neighborhood of the ulcer or by constant support of the tissues by the use of firm elastic bandages over the ulcerated area in the remainder of the leg.

(b) Complete bed rest with daily dressings of a fungicidal powder, plus boric acid ointment is the most effective method of healing.

(3) Rupture of varicose veins.

(a) An occasional complication of varicose veins which may come on suddenly. Easily controlled by elevation of the leg and application of pressure by a tight bandage. Subsequent treatment should be injections of the vein with sclerosing solution or operative resection if this is unsuccessful.

BIBLIOGRAPHY

Heyerdale, W. W., and Stalker, L. K.: 'The Management of Varicose Veins of the Lower Extremities,' *Proc. Staff Meet., Mayo Clin.*, 1941-16-827.

Waugh, J. M.: 'Ligation and Injection of Great Saphenous Veins,' *Proc. Staff Meet., Mayo Clin.*, 1941-16-832.

Weisman, R. E., and Heyerdale, W. W.: 'The Use of a Preliminary Test Dose and the Technic for Injection of Varicosities of the Lower Extremities,' *Proc. Staff Meet., Mayo Clin.*, 1941-16-821.

XVIII

THROMBOPHLEBITIS

A. Etiology.
1. May be a complication of varicose veins.
2. Usually sudden onset, disabling but rarely resulting in embolism.

B. Treatment.
1. In severe cases rest in bed with leg elevated.
2. Application of a wet dressing of boric acid solution.
3. In less extensive cases injections of the uninvolved veins at the periphery of phlebitic area is usually successful.
4. Heparin therapy where indicated.

Iliofemoral Thrombophlebitis (Phlegmasia alba dolens)

A. Etiology.
1. Usually follows abdominal operations or pregnancy.

B. Treatment.
1. Rest in bed until the acute process has subsided. May result in pulmonary embolism.
2. Long standing cases in which the acute process has subsided, characterized by persistent swelling of the lower extremities, may be improved by the use of Buerger's exercises, short wave diathermy and hot sitz baths.
   a. This treatment is not for the acute process.

BIBLIOGRAPHY

Homans, J.: *Circulatory Diseases of the Extremities,* The Macmillan Co., 1939.

XIX

DISEASES OF THE LYMPHATICS OF THE EXTREMITIES

Congenital

A. Simple Lymphangioma.
1. This is a soft, doughy, subcutaneous swelling which may occur on the extremities or on any other part of the body.
2. Usually not tender and is easily compressible.
   a. Treatment.
      (1) Surgical excision in one piece is sometimes possible.
      (2) For the smaller tumors electrocoagulation or radiotherapy may be tried.

B. Cavernous Lymphangioma.
1. As a rule these are large localized swellings which may be multiple and cause peculiar deformities of the extremities.
2. If the overlying skin is very thin they may be punctured easily and exude serous fluid for long periods of time.
3. They may be associated with tumors of the blood vessels thus adding to the difficulties of treatment.
   a. Treatment.
      (1) Unsatisfactory.
      (2) Excision may be tried but is usually unsuccessful as considerable bleeding may be encountered which may be difficult to control.
      (3) Where large areas of an extremity are involved amputation of the entire limb may be the only method of treatment.

Obstruction to the Lymphatic Supply of the Extremities

A. Elephantiasis.
1. In the arm a sequence of radical mastectomy.
2. Treatment of this condition is unsatisfactory.
3. Elephantiasis of lower extremities may be produced by filaria.

B. Milroy's Disease.
1. Congenital familial elephantiasis.
2. May first show itself during puberty.
    a. Treatment is palliative.

C. Sporadic Elephantiasis.
1. Usually affects females more than males.
2. Appears about the time of puberty.
3. Usually found in one leg only but may be bilateral.
4. In many cases it is probably caused by repeated attacks of lymphangitis due to a fungus infection of the feet associated with sudden onset of high temperature and chills.
    a. These attacks may recur over a period of years resulting in chronic swelling of the leg.
    b. Treatment is symptomatic.

BIBLIOGRAPHY

Allan, E. V., and Hines, Jr., E. A.: 'Lipedema of the Legs: A Syndrome Characterized by Fat Legs and Orthostatic Edema,' *Proc. Staff Meet., Mayo Clin.,* 1940-15-184.

Homans, J.: 'Lymphedema of Limbs,' *Arch. Surg.,* 1940-40-232.

Macey, H. B.: 'A New Surgical Procedure for Lymphedema of the Extremities: Report of a Case,' *Proc. Staff Meet., Mayo Clin.,* 1940-15-49.

Pratt, G. H.: 'Surgical Considerations in the Treatment of Chronic Lymphedema and of Varicose Veins,' *Bull., N. Y. Acad. Med.,* June, 1940-381.

GENERAL BIBLIOGRAPHY

Buerger, L.: *Circulatory Disturbances of the Extremities,* W. B. Saunders Co., 1924.

Cowdry, E. V.: *Arteriosclerosis,* The Macmillan Co., 1938.

Diez, J.: *La Tromboangeitis Obliterante,* Buenos Aires, 1934.

Haimovici, H.: *Les Embolies Arterielles des Membres,* Paris, Masson, 1930.

Holman, E.: *Arteriovenous Aneurysm,* The Macmillan Co., 1937.

Homans, J.: *Circulatory Diseases of the Extremities,* The Macmillan Co., 1939.

Kramer, D. W.: *Peripheral Vascular Disorders,* Blakiston, 1940.

Lewis, T. Sir: *Vascular Disorders of the Limbs,* The Macmillan Co., 1937.

The Blood Vessels of the Skin and Their Responses, London, Shaw & Sons, 1927.

Löhr, W.: *Wundheiling,* Leipzig, Barth, 1937.

Mahorner, H. R.: *Thrombo-angiitis Obliterans* (Brown, Allan & Mahorner), W. B. Saunders Co., 1928.

McKittrick, L. S., and Root, H. F.: *Diabetic Surgery,* Lea & Febiger, 1928.

McPheeter and Anderson: *Injection Treatment of Varicose Veins and Hemorrhoids,* Davis, 1939.

Samuels, S. S.: *The Diagnosis and Treatment of Diseases of the Peripheral Arteries* (second edition), Oxford University Press, 1940.

Winternitz, M. C., Thomas, R. M., and LeCompte, P. M.: *The Biology of Arteriosclerosis,* Chas. C. Thomas, 1938.

INDEX

[83]

INDEX

INDEX

OXFORD MEDICAL OUTLINE SERIES

PUBLISHED

IN PREPARATION